UNDERSTANDING diabetes

UNDERSTANDING diabetes

Managing your life
with diabetes

**THE DIABETES CENTRE
ST VINCENT'S HOSPITAL, SYDNEY**

UNDER THE CARE OF THE SISTERS OF CHARITY

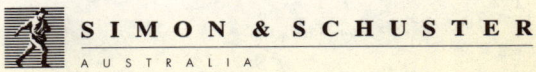

UNDERSTANDING DIABETES

First published in Australia in 1997 by
Simon & Schuster (Australia) Pty Limited
20 Barcoo Street, East Roseville NSW 2069

Reprinted in 2001

A Viacom Company
Sydney New York London Toronto Singapore

Text © St Vincent's Hospital, Sydney, 1997

All rights reserved. No part of this publication may be reproduced, stored in a retrieval system, or transmitted, in any form or by any means, electronic, mechanical, photocopying, recording or otherwise, without the pi permission of the publisher in writing.

National Library of Australia
Cataloguing-in-Publication data

Understanding diabetes : managing your life with diabetes

    Includes index.
    ISBN 0 7318 0551 8.

    1. Diabetes – Popular works. I. St Vincent's Hospital (Sydney, N.S.W.). Diabetes Centre

616.462

Design by Mango Design Group
Printed in Australia by Griffin Press

10 9 8 7 6 5 4 3 2

CONTENTS

Introduction — vii

Chapter 1
What is Diabetes? Why Do You Get It? — 1

Chapter 2
Principles of Diabetes Management — 8

Chapter 3
Achieving Good Diabetes Control: Why and How — 12

Chapter 4
Assessment of Diabetes Control — 16

Chapter 5
Introduction to Food — 23

Chapter 6
Let's Go Shopping — 34

Chapter 7
Exercise — 51

Chapter 8
Insulin Delivery — 58

Chapter 9
Insulin Therapy in IDDM — 65

Chapter 10
Medication in NIDDM — 72

Chapter 11
Hypoglycaemia — 81

Chapter 12
The Highs of Diabetes — 89

Chapter 13 **Avoiding Long Term Complications**	96
Chapter 14 **Foot Care**	104
Chapter 15 **Fertility and Pregnancy**	110
Chapter 16 **Contraception and Hormone Replacement Therapy**	118
Chapter 17 **Sexuality and Diabetes**	121
Chapter 18 **Stress and Diabetes**	140
Chapter 19 **The Adolescent Years**	148
Chapter 20 **Diabetes and the Elderly**	153
Chapter 21 **Eating Away From Home**	162
Chapter 22 **Who Should Be Told?**	170
Chapter 23 **Travel and Diabetes**	174
Chapter 24 **Research in Diabetes**	184
Conclusion	188
Resources	189
Glossary	199
Index	201

INTRODUCTION

Understanding Diabetes is a valuable resource for people with diabetes who want to be fully informed about the latest trends in diabetes care.

Whilst diabetes can add a challenge to many daily activities, the information in this book allows you to plan how better to conduct your life with diabetes successfully. As you are the person most affected by diabetes, you are the key player in managing your life. A variety of health professionals, including your G.P. and the diabetes educators and specialists from the local diabetes service, are all available to help you. By having a sound knowledge base through reading this valuable resource you will be in a better position to minimise diabetes related problems and to maximise life's pleasures.

Lesley Campbell
Judy Reinhardt
The Diabetes Centre
St Vincent's Hospital, Sydney

Acknowledgment:

We wish to thank the following authors for their valuable contribution to the book:

Ms Melissa Armstrong
Sr Wendy Bryant
Assoc Professor Lesley Campbell
Dr Simon Chalkley
Professor Donald Chisholm
Dr Tom Cromer
Dr Brendan Daly
Dr Barbara Depczynski
Mr Tony Diment
Sr Julie Gale
Ms Julia Hill
Dr Tania Markovic
Sr Penny Morris
Dr Margaret Redelman
Sr Judy Reinhardt
Dr Kathy Samaras

Also thanks to Anne-Marie Tannebek for typing of the manuscript and for compiling the chapter on Resources, and thanks to Mrs Pam Morris for proof-reading the manuscript.

Chapter 1

What is Diabetes? Why Do You Get It?

The words *diabetes mellitus* are from the Greek meaning 'sweet urine' — in other words, urine with sugar in it. In today's terms, diabetes mellitus is defined by the presence of a high level of glucose (sugar) in the blood. This chapter describes how the different forms of diabetes develop and how much that development is due to inherited factors.

HOW IS THE BLOOD GLUCOSE LEVEL NORMALLY CONTROLLED?

Sugar comes from the food we eat — either simple sugars or complex carbohydrates — and is absorbed from the intestine after a meal. In between meals, the sugar supply to the bloodstream comes from the liver, which is able to release glucose from its stores or to manufacture it from protein; the storage form of sugar in the liver is glycogen.

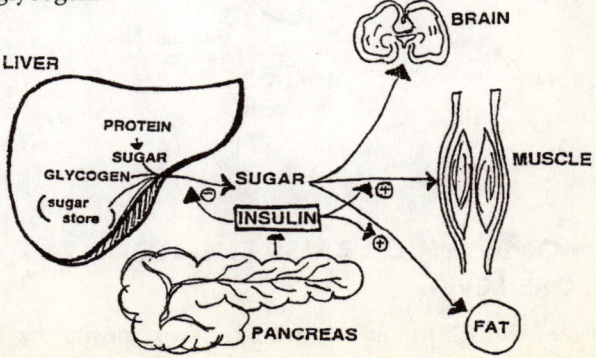

Sugar is needed to keep the brain alive and functioning well and is also used by muscle for energy or by fat cells which can convert sugar to fat stores.

WHAT DOES INSULIN DO?

Insulin is a protein hormone. It is the main factor in controlling a person's blood glucose level. It is produced in relatively large amounts by the islet cells of the pancreas when a meal is eaten or if the blood glucose level is high. In between meals, the islet cells produce a low level of insulin, in order to keep the correct balance between the amount of sugar the liver produces and the use of sugar by the brain, muscles, etc.

The high levels of insulin present when a meal is eaten stop the liver releasing sugar into the bloodstream and help the liver to take up sugar to store as glycogen. Insulin also helps muscle and fat cells to use glucose, which may be used immediately for energy or stored for later needs. These effects of insulin on the liver and other tissues tend to lower the blood glucose level.

The way insulin works to help a muscle cell use glucose is similar to the way a key fits into a lock. The lock opens a door for glucose to pass into the cell. In addition to operating the 'door', insulin also activates proteins (enzymes) in the cell which help the cell either to store glucose as glycogen or use it for energy.

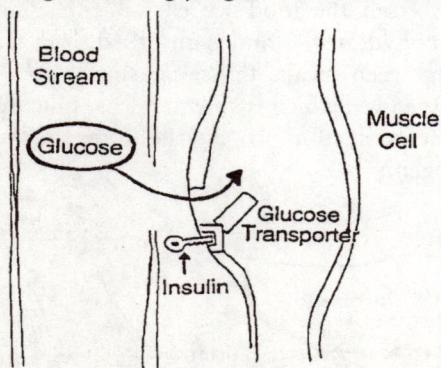

HORMONES WHICH RAISE THE BLOOD GLUCOSE LEVEL

There are several hormones which have the opposite effect to that of insulin and raise the blood glucose level. These work by making the liver put more sugar into the bloodstream. These hormones include glucagon, cortisone and adrenaline. They are sometimes called *stress hormones* because they are useful in making more glucose available for energy during stressful times.

WHAT CAUSES HIGH BLOOD GLUCOSE LEVELS?

In the non-diabetic person, the blood glucose level stays between 3 and 7 mmol/L. There are many problems which can lead to a failure to control the blood glucose level and the development of diabetes. The two most common are:

1. Destruction of the insulin-producing cells by the body's immune system. This causes insulin dependent diabetes mellitues (type 1, juvenile onset); and
2. Poor response of the body to insulin, called insulin resistance. This, together with sluggish insulin production from the islet cells, causes non-insulin dependent diabetes mellitus (type 2, maturity onset).

However, a variety of other problems can cause diabetes. For example:

- damage or destruction of the whole pancreas, e.g. by inflammation (chronic pancreatitis), cancer or iron storage disease (haemochromatosis);
- a rare genetic defect in the insulin molecule or in the lock; or
- rare tumours producing hormones that make the blood glucose level rise (adrenaline or cortisone).

More than 95% of all people with diabetes have one of two types of diabetes: either insulin dependent diabetes or non-insulin dependent diabetes.

WHAT IS INSULIN DEPENDENT DIABETES?

Insulin dependent diabetes mellitus (IDDM) is due to a disturbance of the body's immune system which, over a period of years, destroys the insulin-producing cells of the pancreas, called beta cells (*see* chapter 24, 'Research in diabetes mellitus'). The person feels perfectly well and has no idea that this process is going on until about 90% of the insulin-producing cells are destroyed. The blood glucose level then rises quickly and the person soon becomes unwell.

This type of diabetes can occur at any age, but is most common in the young (under the age of 25) and those who are thin or of normal weight. Insulin dependent diabetes accounts for about 10% of all cases of diabetes.

WHAT IS NON-INSULIN DEPENDENT DIABETES?

Non-insulin dependent diabetes mellitus (NIDDM) is due to a defect in the body's response to insulin. It is as though the lock (which the key, insulin, is operating) is rusty. There is also a sluggishness of the insulin-producing cells — they continue to produce insulin, but not as much as is needed to cope with the rusty lock. These two defects develop gradually until, in middle or older age, the blood sugar rises above normal. The increase in blood glucose levels is often so gradual that it is not noticed. People with this type of diabetes may be unaware of it and may have high blood glucose levels for several years before a diagnosis is made.

Although NIDDM usually has its onset in the middle or older age group, this form of diabetes occasionally occurs in teenagers or young adults. Such people are classified as having maturity onset diabetes of the young (MODY); they usually have a strong family history of NIDDM, but their diabetes usually leads a relatively benign course and they may never progress to a need for insulin treatment. Several different genetic defects of enzymes involved in insulin production or action have now been identified as causes of MODY.

HOW DO PEOPLE KNOW THAT THEY HAVE DIABETES?

In young people with IDDM, symptoms are usually dramatic. The high sugar level in the blood leads to a 'spilling over' of sugar through the kidneys into the urine. The sugar passing through the kidneys drags extra water with it, so that large amounts of urine are produced. As a result, the person urinates a lot and feels dry and thirsty, then drinks a lot. The loss of large amounts of sugar in the urine lowers the body's energy stores and may cause loss of weight, tiredness and a general feeling of being unwell.

High sugar levels may also cause a slight swelling of the lens of the eye which results in blurred vision. This does not indicate any damage to the eye and will get better after the blood glucose level has been controlled. However, the blurring of vision often gets worse for a few days after the diabetes is treated and may take 3–6 weeks to go away. It is best *not* to get new glasses during this period as they are likely to be of the wrong strength.

As a result of the lack of insulin, the liver releases excessive amounts of sugar into the bloodstream, and also produces an excess of ketones (acids) from breaking down the body fat stores. The ketones can cause vomiting and, if present in large amounts, can make the person dangerously ill. This condition of *ketoacidosis* needs emergency treatment with insulin and intravenous fluids (*see* chapter 12, 'The highs of diabetes', for additional information on ketoacidosis).

High sugar levels in the blood also reduce the function of white cells and the immune system, which are responsible for fighting infection. So, people who have developed diabetes and have a high blood glucose level are prone to infection, especially Monilia, (also called thrush), which may affect the genital area, fingernails or mouth.

People with NIDDM usually have less dramatic symptoms. In fact, the symptoms may be so mild that they are disregarded for months or years. Nevertheless, increased passing of urine, thirst, blurred vision and some loss of weight can also occur in NIDDM. Infections, especially with Monilia (thrush), are a very common problem. People with NIDDM generally do not break down fat and suffer from an overproduction of ketones, so they do not usually get as seriously ill as people with IDDM. Occasionally, however, people who have developed NIDDM can slowly develop an extremely high blood glucose level. This can cause severe dehydration so that they, too, become critically ill with hyperosmolar coma. They usually need intravenous fluids and some insulin to recover from this state.

HOW IS THE DIAGNOSIS OF DIABETES MADE?

Not uncommonly, the diagnosis of NIDDM is made following a blood sugar test done at a routine check-up in people who are overweight or have a family history of diabetes. Finding glucose in a urine sample suggests that there may be diabetes, but a blood sugar test must always be done to make a definite diagnosis.

When people are complaining about thirst, blurred vision or other symptoms, their blood glucose level is usually above 11 mmol/L and a single blood sample for a blood glucose level is sufficient to make the diagnosis. In this case, any further tests are usually unnecessary to diagnose diabetes.

If, however, a single blood glucose level is in the borderline range, it may be necessary to perform a glucose tolerance test to make the diagnosis. In this case, the person eats nothing after midnight and has a drink with a lot of glucose in it early in the morning. A blood glucose level is usually taken before the drink and at 1–hour and 2–hour intervals after the drink (sometimes a blood sample is taken every half hour and/or for up to 3 hours).

DID I INHERIT MY DIABETES AND CAN I PASS IT ON TO MY CHILDREN?

The answer to this question is different, depending on whether you are discussing IDDM or NIDDM.

Insulin dependent diabetes (IDDM)

This type of diabetes is not inherited, but there are inherited susceptibility factors. In other words, you inherit a risk of developing IDDM, but environmental 'trigger' factors are necessary to set off the process. These trigger factors are not yet fully understood, but it is quite likely that virus infections may be important. The trigger factors activate a process which continues for years before the diabetes becomes obvious.

Your children will not inherit diabetes and will not be born with diabetes — however, they could inherit a risk of developing the disorder. The chance that the child of someone with IDDM will actually develop diabetes is only about 1 in 30 (the chances are a little higher if a father has diabetes and a little lower if a mother has diabetes). Diet and exercise do not have much influence on whether people get IDDM (although they are important in the treatment of diabetes).

Non-insulin dependent diabetes (NIDDM)

The genetic or inherited contribution to the development of NIDDM is very much stronger than for IDDM — even though the disorder may not occur until later in life. Although the genetic influence for NIDDM is very strong, environmental factors such as diet, exercise and weight control have a major influence on the severity of the disorder. Therefore, people who have the genes for

NIDDM may develop it severely in their forties or fifties if they have a poor diet, are overweight and do not exercise much; whereas they may develop NIDDM mildly in their seventies or eighties if they eat sensibly, exercise a lot and keep to an ideal weight.

WHAT IS THE DIFFERENCE IN APPROACH TO TREATMENT OF IDDM AND NIDDM?

For the first year or two after diagnosis, people with IDDM often find it easy to achieve good control of blood glucose levels with fairly small doses of insulin. This 'honeymoon period' is when there are still some insulin-producing cells functioning in the pancreas. Unfortunately, as time passes these remaining cells fail to survive and there is no supply of insulin other than the insulin which is injected. From this time, blood sugar control requires a careful balance between insulin injections and carbohydrate in the diet. Forgetting a dose of insulin results in a large rise in blood sugar and excessive production of ketones.

People with NIDDM can often control their blood glucose level with weight control and exercise for a substantial period of time. However, as the years go by and the diabetic condition progresses, they often need tablets which help the pancreas produce extra insulin and help the body respond better to insulin. Eventually, as more time goes by, in some people, the insulin-producing cells of the pancreas may become so 'sluggish' that insulin injections are required. Even when this happens, the pancreas usually continues to produce some insulin so blood glucose levels are usually easier to control than in IDDM — and a missed insulin injection will not cause such a serious metabolic disturbance as would occur in IDDM.

It is important to mention that good control of the blood glucose level is equally crucial in both type 1 and type 2 diabetes in order to avoid damage to eyes, kidneys and nerves (*see* chapter 13, 'Avoiding long-term complications').

Chapter 2

Principles of Diabetes Management

Often, when the diagnosis of diabetes is made, people are concerned that their lifestyle may have to change greatly. It is certainly true that having diabetes may compel people to take care of themselves. This chapter outlines the basis for good management of diabetes. The main goals in diabetes care are to improve and/or maintain good health and to lead a life as full and as enjoyable as one could wish.

The basic principles in diabetes care are eating regular balanced meals, undertaking regular physical activity and, when necessary, taking medication. These three principles form the essential elements of the diabetes triangle shown below.

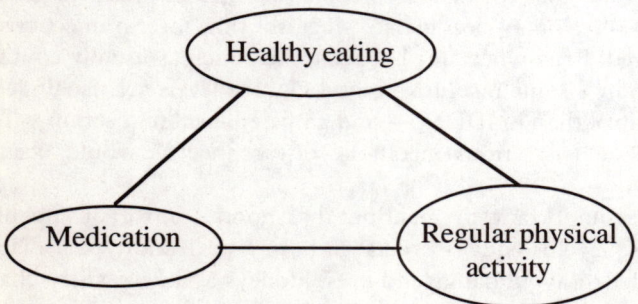

In combination, these three elements are necessary for maintaining or improving health once diabetes is diagnosed. Eating healthy foods and participating in regular physical activity are relevant to the whole community and not only to those with diabetes.

People with insulin dependent diabetes (IDDM) need insulin as part of their regular treatment. On the other hand, people with non-insulin dependent diabetes (NIDDM) often manage at first without any medication. Tablets are usually needed eventually, however, and there are two types: sulfonylureas and metformin. Occasionally, tablets fail to keep the blood glucose levels controlled and then insulin treatment is required for treating people with NIDDM.

As people age, particularly those with NIDDM, there is a greater risk of common problems such as heart disease, raised blood pressure and raised blood fat levels (cholesterol and triglycerides). After the diagnosis of diabetes, more regular checks need to be kept on these and other associated problems to minimise these risks.

SO WHAT DOES ALL THIS MEAN FOR ME?

The first step is to take control of your own health. The essential goal in managing diabetes is to find a good balance between leading a full and active life and having the best possible control of diabetes.

WHAT DOES 'BEST CONTROL' MEAN?

People often think that controlling diabetes means getting the blood glucose levels under a certain level. Obviously, this is an important goal. Keeping blood glucose levels in a healthy range will decrease the chances of developing some of the conditions associated with diabetes that can affect certain parts of the body, such as eyes, kidneys and feet. The best way of achieving ideal glucose levels is through balancing the eating of healthy foods, regular physical activity and medication. While the non-diabetic person will always have a blood glucose level between 3 and 7 mmol/L, people with diabetes are usually advised to keep the blood glucose level between 3 and 7 mmol/L before meals and below 10 mmol/L after meals.

However, there is more to treating diabetes successfully than merely monitoring and maintaining blood glucose levels. Striving to gain 'best control' means looking after all aspects of health. These include blood fat levels, blood pressure and weight. If you follow a healthy diet and undertake regular physical activity, your blood fat levels, blood pressure and weight will usually improve or be maintained. Sometimes, additional treatment may be necessary, such as increasing physical activity to lose weight or taking medication for blood pressure. By looking after these aspects of health care, the risk of some of the problems associated with ageing and diabetes can be avoided or minimised.

WHAT ABOUT MY PSYCHOLOGICAL HEALTH?

When diabetes is diagnosed, people can go through a number of reactions ranging from disbelief to trepidation. Often, doctors and diabetes educators ask people with diabetes to make changes to their lifestyles. These changes may have been attempted before, but, for many reasons, may not have been lasting.
Here are some examples:
- 'I can't believe this is happening to me.'
- 'That can't be right, are you sure?'
- 'This is not really happening to me.'
- 'All these changes will make my life miserable.'

These are a just a few of the many normal reactions experienced. These normal reactions show denial, anger, frustration. Talking about your feelings with your partner, an understanding relative or friend, a doctor or an educator may help. Many people find talking to other people with diabetes helpful, such as in a support group.

Stress is a normal response to many situations. When this is added to the existing stress of a busy life with family, work and social commitments, it is not surprising that stress levels worsen. Sometimes, too much stress can interfere with achieving things that are important. We can become irritable and short-tempered, making it difficult even for sympathetic family members to help. It can be more difficult to carry out important healthy lifestyle changes to improve control of diabetes.

Sometimes there are so many other things to do that achieving or maintaining good health becomes a lower priority. It is very easy to get distracted by the demands of work, family or a busy social life. With diabetes, sometimes it is necessary to be reminded that good health is vital so that one can get on with enjoying the pleasurable parts of life again.

I AM IN CHARGE OF MY HEALTH

When diabetes is diagnosed and lifestyle changes are suggested and medications prescribed, some people feel that they have lost the control of their own health. Most diabetes educational information is aimed at providing people with skills and knowledge to manage their diabetes and to return to them the control of their own health. Health professionals are there to help and advise people with diabetes so that they can manage their disorder. Ideally, when people are the managers of their own health, they also take responsiblity for their own care and seek assistance of health professionals when required.

HOW CAN I IMPROVE MY CONTROL?

Ask yourself the following questions:
- Do I know as much as I can about diet and exercise?
- Am I following my diet and exercise program?
- Am I taking my medication as prescribed?

It may be that finding out a little more information about your diabetes or discussing the advice given by your doctor or educator may help improve your control.

There are times when, even if you are doing everything as suggested, it is possible to lose good blood glucose control. Often, there is a temporary cause: an infection or illness, or the stopping of regular exercise. Occasionally, there is no obvious reason. Whatever the case, additional advice and information should be sought at these times as there is usually a solution.

When diabetes control fluctuates, adjustment of medication may be needed. Insulin doses may have to be adjusted if blood glucose readings are too high or too low. Gaining knowledge about diabetes medications will help you to make simple, small and safe changes to your dose. Your doctor and/or diabetes educator can answer any questions you may have about your medication.

Having diabetes is just one part of life. A few people let it control their lives completely, but this should not be the case. A healthy approach to having diabetes is to know as much as possible about the condition and how it can affect you. You also need to be as active as possible in maintaining the best possible control of your diabetes, so as to achieve the quality of life you desire.

Chapter 3

Achieving Good Diabetes Control: Why and How

WHY DO I NEED GOOD DIABETES CONTROL?

Long-standing diabetes mellitus can be complicated by small and large blood vessel disease and nerve damage. These complications occur in some, but not necessarily all, people with diabetes. In up to 30% of people with diabetes, small vessel disease may show itself as eye and kidney complications. In essence, whether or not people with diabetes get these small vessel complications or nerve damage is related to how well controlled their blood glucose levels are together with their genetic susceptibility to developing these complications. For large vessel disease (e.g. coronary arteries), there may be a lesser connection with how good the blood glucose control is. However, it is largely due to the other known major risk factors for coronary artery disease, such as smoking, high blood pressure, abnormal amounts of lipids (fats) in the blood (cholesterol, triglycerides, etc.) and a family history of coronary heart disease.

Diabetes mellitus may affect the eyes in several ways, including cataract formation and glaucoma, and small vessel disease of the eye (called diabetic retinopathy). Small vessel disease of the kidney (called diabetic nephropathy) causes the kidneys to leak small amounts of protein at first. This eventually increases to larger amounts, with a slow deterioration in kidney function. Also, diabetes mellitus may be complicated by nerve damage (neuropathy), most commonly affecting the nerves in the legs, producing numbness or sometimes pain.

There is more detailed information about diabetic complications in chapter 13. For the moment, however, it is necessary to consider the importance of blood sugar control in causing the problems.

Does good blood glucose control reduce the chance of small blood vessel disease (eye and kidney disease) or of nerve damage in diabetes? The answer is yes for people with insulin dependent diabetes mellitus (IDDM) and almost certainly yes for those with non-insulin dependent diabetes mellitus (NIDDM).

These complications in the eyes, kidneys and nerves (retinopathy, nephropathy and neuropathy) have been conclusively and closely linked to blood sugar control. A large study in America called the DCCT (Diabetes Control and Complications Trial) of people with IDDM was conducted over a 5- to 10-year period. It showed that intensive treatment to lower blood glucose levels reduced the rate of appearance of eye disease (diabetic retinopathy) and kidney disease (diabetic nephropathy) or slowed the progression of these diseases when they were already present. No matter what the starting level of blood sugar was, some improvement in blood glucose level produced a significant reduction in risk or progression of small vessel disease or neuropathy.

About 85–90% of people with diabetes in Australia have NIDDM, while the remainer have IDDM. The obvious question to ask is can the results for the DCCT translate to people with NIDDM? The answer is probably yes and this is supported in a position statement by The Australian Diabetes Society in 1993.

In the DCCT study, large vessel disease (atherosclerosis) manifesting as coronary artery (heart) disease, strokes and impaired circulation to the legs was not affected by better control. Some may argue that this was because this study used only young subjects and coronary artery disease may take longer to appear than the length of the study at the age of the subjects (13 to 39 years old). In people with NIDDM, better blood glucose control has been linked to less coronary artery disease risk in one study of elderly patients and in another study of women. For the moment, it is not known definitely whether or not there is some beneficial effect of good blood sugar control on atherosclerosis.

In addition to trying to improve blood sugar control, people with diabetes should look at any factors that may increase the risk of developing arterial disease. Having NIDDM increases the risk of coronary artery disease by at least twice in men compared to those without it. The addition of any other major risk factor for coronary artery disease, such as smoking, high blood pressure and abnormal blood lipids, further increases the risk. In non-diabetic women who have not yet reached menopause, the female hormones lower their risk of coronary artery disease compared to men of similar age. However, after women reach menopause, the incidence of coronary artery disease catches up to that of men. Women with NIDDM do not enjoy the protective effects of their female hormones on coronary artery disease risk; premenopausal women with diabetes have the same chance of coronary artery disease as men of a similar age.

To reduce the risk of coronary artery disease, people with diabetes (NIDDM and IDDM) should pay special attention to the known additional risk factors for coronary artery disease. It is possible to reduce these risks by changes in lifestyle and/or with use of drug therapy (*see* chapter 13, 'Avoiding long-term complications').

HOW DO I ACHIEVE GOOD DIABETES CONTROL?

The cornerstones of the treatment of NIDDM are diet and exercise, both of which improve blood sugar control. Weight loss and calorie restriction improve blood glucose levels. Exercise alone can improve blood glucose level, blood pressure and blood fat levels, and can help to keep weight down. However, tablets may still be needed eventually to control blood glucose levels or for some people, insulin injections may be required if tablets are no longer effective.

Monitoring blood glucose levels acts as a guide to altering therapy and achieving good blood glucose level control. Simply monitoring urine for the presence of glucose is not enough, as glucose may not appear in the urine until it is well above the blood levels which cause eye and kidney disease and nerve damage. Monitoring blood glucose levels can be done at home by using a drop of blood obtained from a finger pricked by a lancet. This drop of blood is placed on a strip which reacts with the sugar in the blood to produce a change in colour. The blood glucose level is determined from the colour obtained, which can be estimated by eye or more precisely in a glucose meter (*see* chapter 4, 'Assessment of diabetes control').

People with IDDM generally need two or more injections of insulin per day. Four injections usually give better control than two. Frequent monitoring of the blood glucose level makes it easier to achieve optimal control as the insulin dosages can be adjusted with changes in the glucose level.

PHYSICAL EFFECTS OF GOOD BLOOD GLUCOSE CONTROL

In the DCCT study, intensive treatment to improve blood glucose control consisted of taking four or more blood glucose levels a day, and having three or more insulin injections daily or a subcutaneous insulin infusion pump, together with review and support by a team consisting of a psychologist, a dietitian, a social worker and nurse instructors. Obviously not everyone has access to such support or intensive treatment.

Also, in the DCCT trial there was a threefold increase in severe hypoglycaemia with tighter blood sugar control, as well as weight gain in the order of about 4.6 kg over 5 years. People who have hypoglycaemic unawareness and are prone to severe hypoglycaemia would have an increased susceptibility with tight blood glucose control. The occurrence of severe hypoglycaemia would certainly be unacceptable to many and especially to those who are concerned about maintaining a driver's licence (*see* chapter 11, 'Hypoglycaemia', for more information on this condition).

Children under the age of 13 years with IDDM fall into a special group and were excluded from the DCCT trial. Although they seem to be less susceptible to some effects of poor blood glucose control, severe hypoglycaemia may have detrimental effects on their health and wellbeing.

Ultimately, people have to reach a compromise between achieving the best blood sugar control to prevent or retard the progression of small vessel disease and neuropathy, and preventing unwanted side effects of good glycaemic control such as severe hypoglycaemia.

Chapter 4

Assessment of Diabetes Control

Achieving and maintaining 'good' glycaemic control reduces the risk and severity of long- and short-term diabetes complications. So how do we know if good glycaemic control has been achieved? There are a number of testing methods available:
1. urine glucose;
2. urine ketones;
3. home blood glucose monitoring using visual strips or strips with a meter;
4. glycosylated haemoglobin level (HbA1c);
5. fructosamine level.

In considering which method to use when evaluating diabetes control, one must know the benefits and limitations of each type of test. Often, by combining a number of different tests, a fairly complete picture of glycaemic control can be achieved.

URINE GLUCOSE

Urine glucose testing was the original self-monitoring method available to people with diabetes. This method tests for the presence of glucose in the urine, which would indicate a high blood glucose level. This test is no longer widely used or recommended.

Advantages:
- It is quick, easy and relatively cheap to do.
- This testing method is suitable for those who cannot manage blood glucose monitoring and have no one else to assist with blood testing.

Disadvantages:
- This method is imprecise. Varying 'renal thresholds' for glucose means if urine is found positive, the blood glucose could be anything above 10 mmol/L in most people. Renal threshold is the point at which the kidneys allow glucose to leave the body in urine. Some people have very high renal thresholds for glucose, e.g. elderly people. If someone has a high renal threshold their blood glucose level may be up to 15 mmol/L or more with no sugar in the urine.
- There is no measure of hypoglycaemia (low blood glucose).
- This test estimates the glucose level since the last time urine was passed, not the present blood glucose level.

Acceptable therapeutic levels: Absence of glucose in urine.

URINE KETONES

This test measures ketones in the urine. Ketones can result when the body is metabolising fat. The test is intended for people with insulin dependent diabetes (IDDM). It is when the blood glucose level is raised, i.e. above 15 mmol/L, and/or when the person is symptomatic of hyperglycaemia (high blood glucose), and also during times of illness. Test results may be misleading in cases of kidney disease.

HOME BLOOD GLUCOSE MONITORING

Home blood glucose monitoring is where people test their own blood glucose level at home. Capillary blood is obtained after pricking the finger with a sharp 'needle' called a lancet. A drop of blood is put on a testing strip; after a number of seconds, a result can be read either with a meter or by comparing the test strip colour with a colour scale on the side of the test strip container. Most people with diabetes are encouraged to use this type of testing.

Acceptable blood glucose level: between 4 mmol/L and 10 mmol/L. There are exceptions to this acceptable level — e.g. during pregnancy, the acceptable range is more restricted (*see* chapter 15, 'Fertility and pregnancy').

Why do home blood glucose monitoring?

People monitor their blood glucose levels to find out if their diabetes is being managed well. The amount of glucose in the blood goes up and down all day. By testing the blood glucose level, you will be able to determine if it is staying within the healthy range for most of the time.

Also you can check your blood glucose level:
- to substantiate a feeling that the level is high or low;
- to ascertain the effect of exercise;
- to check the effect of a variation in type or quantity of food;
- to see the effects of change in insulin or tablet doses; or
- if you are sick.

There are two ways of estimating your blood glucose level. Both involve pricking the finger to get a drop of blood.

Using visual blood glucose testing

Advantages

- This method is more accurate than urine testing.
- It will show hypoglycaemia and hyperglycaemia.
- Results are often adequate for people with non-insulin dependent diabetes (NIDDM).
- It is a relatively inexpensive test when strips are obtained with NDSS (National Diabetes Services Scheme) assistance.

Disadvantages

- The method relies on people having a satisfactory blood testing technique (poor testing technique will give inaccurate results). While testing your glucose is a fairly easy task, it pays to have your technique checked to make sure you are getting accurate results.
- This technique relies on reasonable eyesight as colours must be compared on a colour scale.
- This method is inappropriate for people with colour blindness.
- The colour scale provides only an estimate, e.g. 9–11 mmol/L, or 11–17 mmol/L. This level of accuracy may be insufficient for some people.

Using reflectance meters and sensors

Advantages
- This technique is easy and more exact than using visual strips.
- This method will show hypoglycaemia and hyperglycaemia.
- The method does not rely on colour vision and may be more easily read by those people with poor vision.
- It is the preferred method for people using insulin and for those with diabetes in pregnancy.

Disadvantages
- As with the visual testing method, this method relies on people having a satisfactory blood testing technique (poor testing technique will give inaccurate results). While testing your glucose is a fairly easy task, it pays to have your technique checked to make sure you are getting accurate results.
- Some meters can prove too difficult for some people to use.
- The accuracy of meters needs to be checked regularly, i.e. with control solutions.
- The cost of buying a meter can be prohibitive. Health insurance companies provide reimbursement for meter purchase, to varying amounts depending on level of insurance cover. A receipt and a letter from a medical practitioner is required for reimbursement.

Normal blood glucose levels

Normal blood glucose levels are those between 3.5 and 7.5 mmol/L. Desired blood glucose levels vary according to the various needs and circumstances of people with diabetes — e.g. for gestational diabetes, the desired range is between 3.5 and 7 mmol/L. For many other people with diabetes, 'good control' is considered to be achieved if the blood glucose level is between 4 and 8 mmol/L, with the occasional reading up to 10 mmol/L. For people with 'brittle' IDDM, levels between 4 and 10 mmol/L, with some higher than 10, may be the best that can be achieved. For the elderly and isolated person, slightly higher levels of 6 to 12 mmol/L may be acceptable in reducing the risk of hypoglycaemia.

Frequency of testing

Frequency of testing depends on type and stability of diabetes. People with NIDDM may test once daily at varying times unless they have high or low readings, in which case they would test more often. People with IDDM often test at least daily at varying times, but need to test more often (i.e. four to five times per day) when diabetes is unstable. People with gestational diabetes usually are instructed to test three to four times per day, i.e. after fasting (before breakfast) and 2 hours after main meals for the duration of the pregnancy.

Timing and recording of tests

Blood glucose levels change during the course of each day. Before meals, the levels tend to fall and then rise again after meals. Varying the times of the day when you do your test is strongly recommended. You can choose from the following times:
- before breakfast
- before lunch
- before dinner
- before bed
- 2 hours after breakfast
- 2 hours after lunch
- 2 hours after dinner
- 2 to 3 a.m. (only if night-time hypoglycaemia is suspected).

After doing a test, it is advisable to record your result. By recording your results in a blood glucose diary, you will be able to see the pattern of your diabetes control. This information will help you and your doctor when making decisions about your diabetes management.

Points to remember about blood glucose monitoring

- Make sure you know how to care for your glucose meter. The person selling the meter should provide full instructions, thorough demonstration and opportunity to practice, on how to use and care for your meter.
- Check the 'use by date' of the strips. Strips outside the expiry date and those not stored correctly will provide inaccurate, misleading results.

- When storing strips, keep the lid on their container. They will be spoiled if left exposed to the air.

GLYCOSYLATED HAEMOGLOBIN (HBA1C)

High concentrations of blood glucose cause non-enzymatic addition of glucose to the haemoglobin molecule; this altered molecule is HbA1c. The life span of haemoglobin is 100–120 days. HbA1c provides an index of integrated glucose concentration over the life span of the haemoglobin. The test gives a retrospective long-term estimate of the average blood glucose level over the preceding 3 months (however, the final 6 weeks have the greatest impact on the result). The test is ordered by a doctor about every 3 months.

Normal values

3.6% to 6.3% (Some laboratory methods, however, have slightly different normal ranges.)

Therapeutic levels

3.6% to 7.4% for most people with diabetes. However, for people with IDDM, HbA1c levels less than 6.5% than are difficult to achieve and potentially dangerous — levels of 6.5–7.5% for people with IDDM are often considered 'ideal'.

FRUCTOSAMINE TEST (GLYCOSYLATED ALBUMIN)

This test measures the concentration of glucose attaching to albumin over its life span. This result provides an index of average glucose concentrations over the preceding 2–3 weeks.

SUPPLIES OF SELF-MONITORING EQUIPMENT

Supplies of home blood glucose monitoring equipment can be obtained from local pharmacies or Diabetes Australia (either directly or by post).

National Diabetes Services Scheme

In operation since 1987, the National Diabetes Services Scheme (NDSS) provides a number of subsidised products for people with diabetes who are registered for the scheme. The NDSS is administered by Diabetes Australia, following government guidelines. People wishing to register for the NDSS must complete the NDSS registration form and send it to Diabetes Australia. Registration is provided free of charge. Applicants will receive a NDSS card through the post from Diabetes Australia.

When purchasing NDSS-listed items, such as test strips and syringes, your card must be shown to participating pharmacists or to Diabetes Australia in order to buy the item at the subsidised price. Not all pharmacists participate in this scheme. Please check with Diabetes Australia to determine the participating pharmacists in your local area. Addresses of Diabetes Australia are located in the final chapter of this book. People who are on a pension or who holds a Health Benefits card will obtain a greater subsidy.

Chapter 5

Introduction to Food

As already stated in chapter 2, good nutrition is an important part of diabetes management. In this chapter, the information given is the latest thinking in regard to the best diet to follow. It is, however, always important to bear in mind that nutrition is a scientific discipline and, for that reason, new research findings may result in a change of advice during a lifetime with diabetes. Perhaps some people reading this book will be surprised at how advice has changed already, even though they may only have been diagnosed with diabetes for a few years.

As more is understood of the theory about what to eat, advice for people with diabetes changes. It is, therefore, a good idea to have contact with a nutrition expert, i.e. dietitian, every couple of years to keep up to date with the latest discoveries. Also, there are many new food products appearing on our supermarket shelves and regular advice can help with keeping up with changes in this area. For individual dietary advice, a general practitioner or endocrinologist can make a referral to a dietitian. Dietitians are found in local hospitals, health care centres and in private practice. The Dietitians Association of Australia can help you find an accredited dietitian in your area.

Everyone with diabetes needs to be assessed individually because of their unique dietary needs. It is not within the scope of this chapter to cover everybody's individual needs, but the basic principles of the dietary management of diabetes will be discussed.

ENERGY

The word energy has many meanings, but, in the nutritional sense, energy is a measure of the fuel that the body needs to function properly. To use an analogy, food is like the petrol in a car. The car cannot run without petrol and the body cannot function without food. Likewise, if the wrong sort of petrol is put into the car, the performance will be affected. If a person eats the wrong food, the same thing will result — poor performance.

The amount of energy the body requires is based on body size, exercise level and age group. Too little energy intake results in weight loss, while excess energy intake causes weight gain. Energy is measured in kilojoules (kJ) in the metric system or in kilocalorie (kCal) in the old imperial system.

Remember everyone is different and there is not a universal energy level.

PROTEIN

Protein is the name given to a particular food component whose role in the body is growth and tissue repair. For example, protein forms new skin to heal a cut. Fingernails, hair and muscle are also made of protein. Very little protein is required in the diet every day because the body recycles much of its protein.

Contrary to what our mothers or grandmothers told us, large amounts of protein are not needed to build big, strong muscles. What is needed is exercise to build the muscles from the protein that is already available. Good food sources of protein are meat, chicken, fish, eggs, cheese, yoghurt, milk, legumes and nuts. These foods also provide essential vitamins and minerals, e.g. thiamine (vitamin B1) and iron. Unfortunately (except for legumes), they are also good sources of fat. See the next chapter on food for more on this point.

FAT

Fat is the part of food which provides the most concentrated energy. If more energy is eaten than is needed, the body stores it as fat for later use. Some body fat is essential. It surrounds and protects important organs such as the kidneys and is also a source of some hormones. Animals, like humans, also store fat and this is why food from animals also contains fat. Fat is present in seeds and nuts to give energy to the new plant when it starts to grow. Fat from food also carries vitamins, e.g. vitamins A, D, E and K, which makes fat an essential part of our diet.

Fat in food is described by its chemical structure as polyunsaturated, monounsaturated and saturated. These different types of fat are found in different proportions in different food. As a general rule, foods that are animal in origin, e.g. meat and dairy food, contain mostly saturated fat. Fats from fruit or vegetable sources, e.g. olives, sunflowers and avocados, contain mono-unsaturated or polyunsaturated fats. Recommendations about which fats to eat follow on page 37.

CARBOHYDRATE

Foods which contain carbohydrate provide the most readily available and preferred source of energy: glucose. Every cell in the body uses glucose. Some tissues, e.g. the brain, use glucose exclusively. As body cells (and we have billions of them) require glucose as a form of energy, it is essential that there is sufficient carbohydrate food in your diet every day to keep the body running efficiently. In fact, it is preferable to have these foods at every meal, i.e. spaced out across the day to provide the body with a steady source of fuel.

Carbohydrate foods are sometimes divided into starches and sugars, but their effects on the body are surprisingly similar to one another. Many carbohydrate-containing foods also contain fibre and are good sources of vitamins.

FIBRE

Fibre is the indigestible part of food which passes right through the digestive system. Fibre helps regulate bowel function and may help protect against bowel cancer. As fibre is not digested, it leaves a feeling of fullness after eating. This can be very useful for those trying to lose weight and who struggle with hunger pangs only 1–2 hours after eating.

When increasing the fibre content of your diet, it is best to do so slowly as increased fibre intake does mean increased gas production in the bowel, resulting in flatulence. If fibre is increased slowly, this problem is less troublesome as the bowel has time to adapt to its new diet.

VITAMINS

The word vitamin is derived from the Latin word vita which means life. Vitamins regulate essential body functions and without them deficiency diseases can develop. They are only needed by the body in small quantities. Some vitamins can be toxic if taken in large amounts, e.g. vitamin A.

Sufficient vitamins can be obtained from eating a wide variety of fruits, vegetables and animal products. Vitamin supplements should only be taken if your diet is inadequate. The majority of Australians do not have vitamin deficiency problems. Recently, it has been recommended that all women contemplating pregnancy should take a daily folic acid supplement to reduce their risk of having a child with a neural tube defect such as spina bifida. If in doubt about your need for a vitamin supplement, discuss this with your dietitian or doctor.

MINERALS

Minerals, like vitamins, are usually needed by the body in small quantities. The exception to this is calcium, which is the main component of bones and teeth. Different foods contain different minerals and so a diet with plenty of variety will provide all the minerals required.

If any of the food groups are avoided, mineral deficiencies may occur, e.g. if dairy foods are avoided completely, the body will not have sufficient calcium to build and maintain strong, healthy bones. Alternative sources of calcium would need to be included in the diet instead.

Dietary guidelines for Australians

The dietary guidelines for people with diabetes are the same as those for all Australian people. The best diet for people with diabetes is also ideal for lowering cholesterol and reducing the risk of some cancers.

The first Australian dietary guidelines were released in April 1979 and were revised in the early 1990s. The revised guidelines were launched by the National Health and Medical Research Council (NHMRC) in 1992.

Dietary guidelines for Australians (1992)

1. Enjoy a wide variety of nutritious food.
2. Eat plenty of breads and cereals (preferably wholegrain), vegetables (including legumes) and fruits.

3. Eat a diet low in fat, particularly saturated fat.
4. Maintain a healthy body weight by balancing physical activity and food intake.
5. Limit alcohol intake.
6. Eat only a moderate amount of food containing added sugars.
7. Choose low-salt food and use salt sparingly.
8. Encourage and support breastfeeding.

Guidelines on specific nutrients

1. Eat food containing calcium. This is particularly important for girls and women.
2. Eat food containing iron. This is especially important for girls, women, vegetarians and athletes.

Dietary guidelines for children

1. Encourage and support breastfeeding.
2. Enjoy a wide variety of nutritious food.
3. Eat plenty of breads, cereals (preferably wholegrain), vegetables (including legumes) and fruits.
4. Low-fat diets are not suitable for children. For older children, a diet low in fat and in particular, low in saturated fat, is appropriate.
5. Maintain a healthy body weight by balancing physical activity and food intake.
6. Water is the preferred drink for children; alcohol is not recommended.
7. Eat only a moderate amount of sugars and food containing added sugars.
8. Choose low-salt food and use salt sparingly.

Guidelines on specific nutrients

1. Eat food containing calcium.
2. Eat food containing iron.

Let's look at each of these points in turn, with some practical advice to help achieve these goals.

1. **Enjoy a wide variety of nutritious food**

   By eating from all the food groups and having a variety of food from those groups adequate intake of vitamins and minerals will be ensured. Conversely, if an entire food group, (e.g. dairy foods) is missed, your total diet will be inadequate — in this example, calcium intake.

2. **Eat plenty of breads and cereals (preferably wholegrain), vegetables and fruit**

   Remember carbohydrates — the body's essential fuel source. The following foods are packed full of carbohydrates: breads, cereals, vegetables and fruit. These should form the basic structure of your diet. They are very low in fat (unless it has been added) and full of fibre, vitamins and minerals.

Wholegrain (unprocessed) cereals contain even more fibre, vitamins and minerals. These food should be eaten at every meal and in quantities to satisfy your appetite.

3. **Eat a diet low in fat and in particular, low in saturated fat**

   When fat is eaten, it makes body fat and cholesterol. When too much fat is eaten, too much body fat and cholesterol can be produced. By eating less fat, you will not add to the body's fat stores, e.g. around the stomach and thighs. Also, by eating less fat, you will significantly reduce the total amount of fuel going into your body (i.e. less kilojoules), which will then help you lose excess weight.

   Add only small amounts of fat-containing foods to the basic structure of breads, cereals, vegetables and fruit. Saturated fats (usually from animal sources) make cholesterol more easily than other fats, so reducing intake of this type of fat is especially important.

4. **Maintain a healthy body weight by balancing physical activity and food intake**

   Body weight is a balance between how much food is eaten and how much exercise is done. Eat more and/or exercise less and body weight increases. Eat less and/or exercise more and your body weight decreases. Obviously, if you are trying to lose weight, a combination of increased exercise and decreased food intake will result in a larger and quicker weight loss. People who increase exercise to help weight loss are most likely to keep weight off. For people who see themselves as 'failed dieters', participating in exercise may be a big help. For more about exercise, see chapter 7, 'Exercise'.

5. Limit alcohol intake

Alcohol contains a large amount of energy (kilojoules/calories) and can contribute to an excess of body fat. Large quantities of alcohol, either daily or in binges, can damage almost every organ in the body. Safe levels of alcohol intake have been suggested by the National Health and Medical Research Council (NHMRC), i.e. less than/equal to 4 standard drinks per day for men and less than 2 drinks per day for women, with one alcohol-free day per week. Women are more susceptible to alcohol damage than men, hence, for safety, women should drink less than men.

A standard drink is:
1 x 120 mL (one glass) of wine = 1 middy beer = 1 schooner of low-alcohol beer = 1 nip (30 mL) spirits = 60 mL fortified wine, e.g. sherry

Refer to chapter 21, 'Eating away from home', for more information on alcohol.

6. Eat only moderate amounts of sugars and food with added sugars

Excessive quantities of sugar will cause large rises in blood glucose levels. Small quantities of sugar have little effect. Keep reading for more information on this relevant subject.

7. Choose low-salt food and use salt sparingly

In susceptible individuals, a large salt intake is linked to high blood pressure. Unfortunately, it is impossible to know who is sensitive and who is not. So, a general guideline has been developed for everyone. Try first adding a little salt into cooking, but leaving that salt shaker in the kitchen so no more is added at the table. Choose salt-free/salt-reduced packaged food where possible.

8. Encourage and support breastfeeding

To simplify, breast is best! Breast milk contains all the nutrition and protective factors a baby needs. Today's infant formulas are good, but nothing beats breast milk.

Specific nutrients

1. **Calcium**

    Calcium has already been briefly mentioned. Women are more likely to suffer osteoporosis (thinning of the bones) than men. However, it has recently been recognised that increasing numbers of men are developing osteoporosis. Therefore, a good calcium intake throughout your life will help to develop strong, healthy bones and ensure peak adult bone mass is achieved. This reduces the risk of developing osteoporosis later in life.

    The major contributors to calcium intake are milk (especially those with added calcium), cheese (low-fat is best), calcium-enriched soy milk and yoghurt (low-fat is best). The following foods contribute small quantities of calcium: dark green, leafy vegetables, sardines and salmon eaten with the edible bones, sesame seeds and tahini (sesame paste), and firm tofu.

2. **Iron**

    Iron helps carry oxygen around the body — what could be more important than that? Women lose iron each month in their regular menstrual cycle, so it is important that this iron is regularly replaced. Red meat is an excellent source of iron, but it is also found in legumes, wholegrain cereals and some vegetables in smaller amounts. Food containing vitamin C, e.g. fruit, helps the body absorb iron, especially from these non-meat sources.

    Athletes have an increased need for iron because of their high level of training. People who eat little or no red meat also need to ensure that they receive an adequate iron intake by eating a wide variety of wholegrain cereals and legumes.

BODY IMAGE AND SHAPE

It is interesting to note that as the ideal female image of beauty grows slimmer over the years, the actual percentage of people in Australia who are overweight or obese is increasing rapidly. According to the most recent Heart Foundation survey, almost 50% of men and almost 40% of women in Australia are overweight or obese.

Most people with NIDDM are overwieght to some degree or perhaps even suffer from obesity. There is much evidence in such people that some weight loss can improve blood glucose levels, blood fat levels and even blood pressure. Thus, a very common aim of diabetes management is to lessen a person's weight.

However, there is much anguish about the subject of weight, partly because a large proportion of the community is 'on a diet' at any given time, trying to lose weight either necessarily or unnecessarily. There is often an unrealistic expectation of what is a healthy weight and fad diets with poor nutritional basis are common.

Recent research suggests that there is a strong genetic influence on how fat (or thin) we are. This does not mean that nothing can be done to lose weight: most chronic disorders we suffer from have some genetic component, but are still able to be treated effectively. Medical research, however, has been very useful in showing us the approaches which do not work (whatever the women's magazines may promise).

Rapid weight loss achieved through crash diets is almost invariably unsuccessful in the long term. This is probably because the body, quite reasonably, senses a famine coming if weight loss is very rapid and, when the strict dieting phase has finished, usually regains the lost weight. Also, the body tends to lose large amounts of muscle tissue as well as fat in this rapid type of weight loss. There may occasionally be medical reasons for needing such a rapid weight loss (an operation or a serious medical condition caused by obesity) and a low-kilojoule diet will be prescribed medically. However, this usually only has a short-term effect unless other measures are taken in the long term. The medical term for this type of diet is the *very low calorie diet* (VLCD). It restricts energy to about 800 calories (2560 kJ) per day. This type of dieting must only be carried out under proper medical supervision in case any complications occur.

Everyone knows that to lose weight, less energy must be taken in than is expended. The clever way to achieve this is to achieve weight loss gradually, by increasing what is expended as well as making some changes to what is taken in. Most doctors now know to give an exercise prescription as well as dietary advice when helping people to lose weight. There has been evidence that the person who loses weight and maintains an increased physical activity will be much more likely to keep that weight off than the person who loses weight by diet only.

For many people, it is difficult to find a suitable form of activity, but it is useful to know that walking is probably the best form of exercise (and the cheapest). The aim is to try to walk briskly for up to an hour or more on 3–5 days of the week. It is safest to start with a short walk and build up slowly, taking care to wear comfortable shoes, see a podiatrist beforehand, if necessary, and check your feet afterwards for signs of damage. Many people find that they can burn more energy in other ways as well: taking the stairs regularly instead of the lift; walking part of the way to and/or from work; buying an active dog; doing some errands on foot; etc. It is best not to weigh yourself frequently to monitor progress, but rather to measure the waist and other areas for loss of centimetres, and to look at the improvement in blood glucose levels, fat levels and blood pressure. During difficult or stressful times, it can be important to maintain weight rather than to gain it. Keeping an exercise regimen going will be good for your health even if no weight loss occurs.

If initial diet and exercise do not achieve satisfactory weight loss, there can be benefit from the use of the appetite suppressant dexfenfluramine (Adifax). It is not a stimulant nor is it addictive as the old amphetamine-style appetite suppressants were. It helps normalise the eating patterns by increasing the feeling of fullness with meals and diminishing the desire for high-energy snacks. Minor side effects include drowsiness and dizziness. In Australia, it is recommended for 3 months' use at a time and, if successful, can be used again at intervals. It must be prescribed and used under a doctor's supervision. It has a particular bonus in people with diabetes, separate to its effect on weight loss, as it tends to improve insulin sensitivity and decrease blood glucose. At present, there are no other safe drugs available for weight loss, but an enormous amount of research work is being done, particularly since the recent discovery of an 'obesity' gene product (in mice) which can make obese mice slim.

Surgery has been used in the past for morbid obesity and its place in medical management is becoming clearer. There have been some barbaric practices which have fallen in to disuse in most places, such as intestinal bypass (causing severe malabsorption of food and diarrhoea) and jaw wiring (to restrain eating physically). Currently, in people with medical complications from severe obesity, an operation to narrow the stomach with staples or a band can result in major weight loss. This is specialised surgery best done in surgical units where it is common. The drawbacks must always be pointed out to the potential patient: it is impossible to eat normally again afterwards unless the operation is reversed. The capacity of the stomach is so small that vomiting can occur with anything more than a cupful of food. There is a need for psychological assessment beforehand as the restriction on normal eating and the large weight loss can have major emotional impacts.

Many people dream of liposuction or a cosmetic surgery procedure draining fat away from the body without any personal effort. The real use of such plastic procedures is to improve the body appearance after weight loss, when redundant skin or lax supporting tissue is trimmed. Any small volumes of fat removed by liposuction will return if lifestyle changes and weight loss do not occur as well. Liposuction can be useful, however, in people who have developed lumpiness at insulin injection sites (*see* chapter 8, 'Insulin delivery').

People with diabetes who need to lose weight should always do so with medical supervision. The changes in exercise and food intake will always need to be taken into consideration in those who take diabetes medication (either tablets or insulin). The risk of hypoglycaemia, from the first days of dietary change, is a real one, even before weight loss occurs. Medication may need to be lowered frequently. Fad diets can be dangerous for diabetic people, e.g. a very low (ketogenic) carbohydrate diet. Also, the impact of exercise on the feet, eyes and blood pressure must all be evaluated before the exercise so that weight loss can be effective, safe and maintained throughout life. Understanding what can be achieved is important so that unrealistic (and unsuccessful) dieting attempts do not occur.

With a concerted long-term approach, weight can be lost and, even more importantly, the weight loss maintained.

Chapter 6

Let's Go Shopping

The basic principles of diet were outlined in the last chapter. Now you need to consider how to put them into practice.

The most important knowledge you need when you hit the supermarket is how to read food labels. If you are able to decipher the information given on the label, you will be able to choose the correct food very easily.

Food labelling is governed by the Australian Food Standards Code. Each state and territory employs food inspectors to check the laws are being complied with by the manufacturers. The Australian New Zealand Food Authority (ANZFA) is responsible for recommending what goes on food labels and what is allowed in food.

WHAT GOES ON A FOOD LABEL?

- The label must be legible, easily visible and in English.
- Nothing false or misleading can be contained on the label.
- The name of the food must be given.
- A list of ingredients in descending order of weight (except water) must be provided.
- Any additives to the food must be listed.
- The country in which the food was made must be given or a statement made that the ingredients are imported.
- The name of manufacturer/importer/packer/vendor must be included.
- Date marking must be used to indicate the food's minimum durable life.
- If a nutrition claim is made, e.g. low-fat, then a nutrition panel must be shown to complement this claim.

Let's Go Shopping

A Code of Practice was introduced by the ANZFA in January 1995 to provide further guidelines for manufacturers when labelling their products. The aim is to provide consumers with consistent information from food manufacturers.

The Code of Practice covers the use of such terms as 'lite/light', 'low-fat', 'reduced fat', 'low in sugar', 'no added sugar' etc. For a copy of this Code of Practice, write to:

Australia New Zealand Food Authority (ANZFA)
PO Box 7186
Canberra MC, ACT 2610
Tel: (02) 6271 2222

What should I look for on labels?

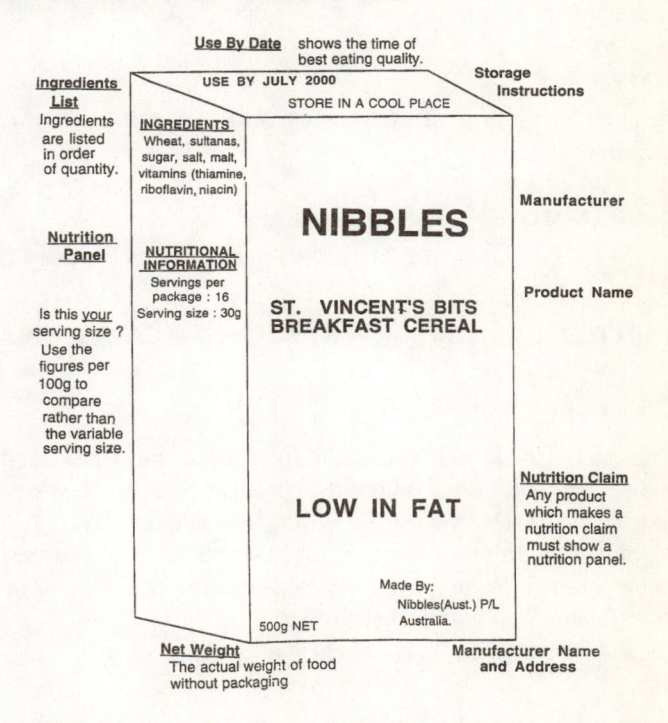

Use By Date shows the time of best eating quality.
USE BY JULY 2000

Storage Instructions
STORE IN A COOL PLACE

Ingredients List
Ingredients are listed in order of quantity.
INGREDIENTS
Wheat, sultanas, sugar, salt, malt, vitamins (thiamine, riboflavin, niacin)

Manufacturer

NIBBLES

Nutrition Panel
NUTRITIONAL INFORMATION
Servings per package : 16
Serving size : 30g

Is this *your* serving size? Use the figures per 100g to compare rather than the variable serving size.

Product Name
ST. VINCENT'S BITS BREAKFAST CEREAL

LOW IN FAT

Nutrition Claim
Any product which makes a nutrition claim must show a nutrition panel.

Made By:
Nibbles(Aust.) P/L
Australia.

500g NET

Net Weight
The actual weight of food without packaging

Manufacturer Name and Address

HOW TO COMPARE BRANDS

By checking the nutrition information under 'per 100 g', it is possible to compare different products even though they come in a varied range of serving sizes.

Fat

Use the figure per 100 g and pick the one with the least fat. Also, look for products with less than 10 g fat per 100 g.

Carbohydrate

Total: This includes sugars and starches. If you are on an 'exchange' or 'portion' diet, you can work out how many 'exchanges' you are eating.
Sugars: This will include added sugars as well as the naturally occurring sugars in milk (lactose) and fruit (fructose). Cross-check with the ingredients list to find the source(s) of sugar. For intance, if a cereal contains sultanas, a higher sugar content is acceptable.

Dietary fibre

Once again use the figure per 100 g and pick the one with the highest fibre.

Sodium (salt)

Where possible, choose products with reduced or no added salt.

NUTRITION CLAIMS – WHAT THEY REALLY MEAN

Lite or light

The characteristic which makes the food 'light' must be stated on the label, e.g. 'light' olive oil is either paler in colour or less strong-tasting than other olive oils. It is not lower in energy (kJ) than other olive oils. In other foods like potato chips, 'lite' can mean a low-salt product. If the term refers to the energy (kJ) content of the food, it must comply with the standards code.

Diet

This term has been used by food companies to imply that the product has a particular nutritional property. It is most often used to describe products whose energy (kJ) content is lower than other similar foods. This usage is now covered by the Food Standards Code to ensure the word 'diet' is always used in this context.

No added sugar

This means no added or additional sugar, e.g. glucose, honey, fructose etc. However, this does not always mean it will contain less energy (kJ) as many foods are naturally high in sugar. Again, cross-check by referring to the nutrition panel.

Cholesterol free

Cholesterol is only found in products of animal origin. For instance, avocados have always and will always be cholesterol free. Importantly, cholesterol free does not mean fat free.

Low-fat

This term can only be used when the food contains less than 3 g fat per 100 g.

Low joule

This term usually means that the food has been artificially sweetened.

No added salt

This term means salt has not been added to the food.

High fibre

The food must contain at least 3 g fibre per average serve.

The National Heart Foundation have developed the 'Pick the Tick' campaign to help people choose low-fat, low-salt food. This can be very helpful when choosing food at the supermarket. However, many suitable foods do not pay to display the NHF tick. With good food label reading skills, it is possible to choose the right foods, tick or no tick.

In the previous chapter, the guidelines for a healthy diet were explained. Following are some practical suggestions to help decrease the fat content of your diet.

ADDED FATS

The fats we add to food are the easy ones to target first. The following are all sources of fat: margarine, butter, oil, cream and sour cream.

Note:
- Margarine, butter and oil all have the same energy content, i.e. 600 kJ (143 kCal) per tablespoon.
- Cream has 280 kJ (67 kCal) per tablespoon.
- Sour cream has 150 kJ (36 kCal) per tablespoon.

Step 1 When choosing which fats to use, the first important point to consider is the source of the fat. Animal fats (or saturated fats), e.g. butter, cream and sour cream, are most closely linked to elevated blood cholesterol levels and should be strictly limited in your diet. Vegetable fats (or polyunsaturated or monounsaturated fats), on the other hand, have a lesser tendency to increase blood cholesterol. However, in excess, they can still cause a rise in cholesterol.

Of course, there are always exceptions to the rule. The fats in fish are unlike those in land-based animals and behave more like vegetable oils. In fact, they may confer some benefit in relation to cardiovascular disease. Coconut oil and palm oil, while coming from plants, are saturated fats and will therefore raise cholesterol in the same manner as animal fats.

Step 2 Having chosen a suitable vegetable fat, use only small quantities each day. Three to four teaspoons per day is enough for most adults.
Example:

> Harold was used to using lots of butter on his toast and in his mashed potatoes. He was surprised to hear the dietitian tell him that his excess fat was contributing to his being overweight and to his cholesterol problem. He hated the taste of margarine. So, as a first step, Harold changed to a half butter/half canola oil spread and reduced the quantity he used. After a few months, he bought a tub of canola margarine and found he did not find the taste too bad. Anyway, by this time he just scraped it thinly on his bread so there wasn't a strong flavour left. He liked the fact that is was easy to spread, too. The dietitian then suggested trying the reduced-fat margarine spread, but enough was enough, and Harold kept with his 3–4 teaspoons of canola margarine per day. Anyway, by that time he had lost

4 kg and his cholesterol had dropped from 7.2 mmol/L to 6.0 mmol/L. He felt very pleased with his success.

HIDDEN FATS

Dairy food

As we learned in the previous chapter, dairy food is an essential element in a healthy, balanced diet. However, this food can add lots of saturated fat to your diet if you do not choose wisely. Luckily, there are lots of low-fat dairy products on the supermarket shelves from which to choose.

Step 1 Choose a low-fat milk. These vary in fat content from state to state, so read the food labels and choose wisely. Some low-fat milks now have added extras such as calcium and iron, making them very beneficial in helping us to meet our daily requirements for these nutrients.

Step 2 Choose low-fat yoghurt. These come as plain or as flavoured yoghurts. The flavoured yoghurts are also available in artificially sweetened versions.

Step 3: Choose a low-fat cheese. Again, label reading skills are invaluable. The low-fat cheeses vary significantly in their fat content. The best ones are those which contain 10 g fat per 100 g or less. Ricotta and cottage cheese are naturally low in fat and easily come in under the magical 10 g limit:
ricotta cheese — 8.2 g fat per 100 g
cottage cheese — 9.5 g fat per 100 g
low-fat cottage cheese — 1.0 g per 100 g
(Note: 'light' cream cheese still has 16 g fat per 100 g and it is saturated fat. Use margarine instead.)

Step 4 Choose low-fat ice cream products. Read the food labels and choose the one with the lowest fat content. Some frozen dessert products are based on fruit and contain no fat at all.

Intolerance to dairy products

A small number of Australians are intolerant of cows' milk and choose a soya milk instead. Again, manufacturers have come to the rescue and have produced a low-fat soya milk. Always choose a soya milk with added calcium, i.e. at least 100 mg calcium per 100 mL soya milk.

Meat, chicken, eggs and fish

Animals and fish, like humans, store excess energy as fat. Therefore, animal and fish foods also contain fat. Some of this fat we can see, such as the thick rind of fat along the edge of a piece of steak or a lamb chop, or the skin of a chicken. However, even when that visible fat is removed there is still hidden fat in the meat. For this reason, choose cuts of meat carefully. **Note:** chicken and red meat have about the same fat content.

Step 1 Choose lean meat, e.g. trim lamb, new-fashioned pork, best mince, skinless poultry.

Step 2 Avoid processed meat such as salami, devon and sausages which contain extra added fat.

Step 3 Eat more fish and seafood. Fish and seafood are much lower in fat than meat and chicken, i.e. about 1% fat. If high cholesterol is a problem, limit shelled seafood, e.g. prawns, lobster and crab, to once a week.

Step 4 Eggs, too, contain fat which is invisible — about 6 g fat (1 teaspoon) in each egg. If cholesterol is elevated, limit eggs to two to three per week.

Step 5 Eat one or two small serves of meat, chicken or eggs per day, eat larger serves of fish. Remember, because these products still contain fat (although invisible), you should be careful about the serving sizes. Fill up with lots of vegetables and carbohydrate food such as rice, pasta or potatoes.

3. Baked goods

Baked goods are another source of hidden fats. All biscuits, cakes and pastries are made with fat. Biscuits can vary greatly in their fat content — both sweet and savoury varieties. As a general rule the more 'plain' the biscuit, the less fat it contains. Compare the biscuits in the following table.

Type of biscuit	Fat per 100 g
Plain, sweet biscuits	16.1 g
Fruit-filled biscuits	3.0–9.9 g
Short bread biscuit	24.9 g
Cream and jam filled biscuits	23.3 g
Chocolate-coated, cream-filled biscuit	28.7 g
Wholemeal crispbread	9.7 g
Flaky cracker	14.3 g
Small, round cracker	23.8 g
Small, flavoured cracker	24.3 g
Water cracker	9.3 g

(Reference: Rosemary Stanton's *Fat and Fibre Counter,* Wilkinson Books, 1993.)

Depending on the type, cake is a high-fat food, too. The majority of pastries (sweet and savoury) are made with large quantities of fat and should be avoided as much as possible. The exception to this is filo pastry.

Type of pastry	Fat per 100 g
flaky	40.0 g
puff	28.0 g
shortcrust	21.5 g
filo	2.9 g

Tip: To keep filo low in fat, brush egg white or skim milk between the layers, rather than melted butter.

Snack foods

Many snack foods contain lots of fat, e.g. nuts, chips, corn chips, chocolate or carob bars. There are many healthier snacks to try, e.g. dried/fresh fruit, bread, low-fat yoghurt, popcorn (without the butter added), Vitari ice cream, etc.

Type of snack food	Fat per 100 g
carob/chocolate	30 g
Cadbury Lite chocolate	28 g
corn chips	25 g
potato chips	36 g
'light' potato chips	26-30 g
macadamia nuts	76 g

MORE INFORMATION ABOUT SUGAR IN YOUR DIET

It is in this area that advice has most changed over the years. Small quantities of sugar do not cause a rapid and uncontrollable rise in blood glucose levels. Very strict avoidance of sugar in a diabetic meal plan is not necessary. Perhaps you have noticed this yourself and it is no real news to you. For others, this may seem like heresy.

This new advice about sugar comes from research which has determined the blood glucose raising effects of many different foods in actual people, including adults with diabetes. We now understand that different carbohydrate-containing foods are digested at different rates and so have different effects on blood glucose levels. This measure of the effect on blood glucose levels is called the *glycaemic index* or GI of a food. These experiments have shown that small quantities of sugar do not cause big rises in blood glucose levels.

The key point here is the quantity of sugar, rather than whether to have sugar or not. For example, it is very sensible to avoid soft drinks and cordials which contain a lot of sugar in a relatively small volume, e.g. there are approximately 11 teaspoons of sugar in each can of lemonade or cola drink. If only one lolly or a small piece of chocolate is eaten, the effect on the blood glucose level is small; if half a packet is eaten, the effect will be large!

Many people with diabetes have deprived themselves of excellent packaged or processed foods in the mistaken belief that 'any sugar is too much sugar'. Dietitians now agree that the majority of breakfast cereals and many biscuits are suitable in a diabetic meal plan. Look for cereals that are low in fat and high in fibre, rather than being too worried about the sugar content. For example:

> Mr N had been an insulin-dependent diabetic for 40 years. At his recent visit to the dietitian, he was pleasantly surprised by the new advice given to him in regard to sugar. He realised that he had been over-restricting his diet for years and missing out on a whole range of delicious products. He would enjoy working his way through the updated list of suitable biscuits and cereals!
>
> It was also nice no longer to feel guilty about the regular scoop of ice cream or the scrape of jam on his Sunday morning scones. He had not noticed that

these foods increased his blood glucose levels, but he had felt guilty nonetheless. He was very happy the GP suggested this return visit to his local diabetes centre.

It is important to remember that although the sugar may not make the blood glucose levels rise, it still contains energy or kilojoules, and this should be taken into consideration when trying to lose weight.

More about the glycaemic index

The glycaemic index (GI) of a food is determined by measuring the actual rise in blood glucose levels after eating a particular food and comparing this to the effect of eating pure glucose. This provides a ranking of foods. Glucose has a ranking of 100 and most other carbohydrate foods are ranked underneath this figure. This has shown us that, within particular foods groups, there may be some foods which are better choices to eat as they may have a more beneficial effect on blood glucose levels. For example, different types of rice or bread (e.g. wholemeal) may cause a slower rise in blood glucose levels. To paraphrase George Orwell: 'all carbohydrates foods are equal, but some are more equal than others.'

It must be remembered, however, that there are still individual variations in blood glucose responses to foods. Some experimentation may be required to determine what is best for you.

There are a few problems associated with the glycaemic index. Assessment of the glycaemic index has not been carried out on children or pregnant women, so we do not know for sure that the same responses will occur in these groups.

There are many commercially available foods which have not been tested. It is hoped that all foods will routinely be tested eventually, but we are a long way from this at the moment. At present, we cannot list all the lowest glycaemic index foods in every food category.

Be wary of taking the glycaemic index value of a food too literally. Just because one piece of fruit has a higher glycaemic index than another, it does not mean it is a 'bad' food. It simply means that you may notice a difference in blood glucose levels after eating different types of fruits. Moreover, when a carbohydrate food of different glycaemic index value is eaten as part of a meal mixed with some protein and fat, the difference in effect on blood glucose levels may be much less than would be predicted from the index.

As yet, no research has been done linking the glycaemic index of a food with its potential for treating a hypoglycaemic episode. Please continue to use the tried and true methods of treating hypos, which are mentioned elsewhere in this book.

The glycaemic index is another one of the tools dietitians use when trying to help each person with diabetes follow the best individualised meal plan for them. This new area of food research is very exciting for everyone involved in diabetes care. Please discuss these issues with your dietitian, diabetes educator or doctor next time you visit to find out the latest good news.

CARBOHYDRATE EXCHANGES OR PORTIONS

Some people have been taught by their dietitian how to count the daily carbohydrate content using an exchange or portion diet system. This is especially useful for anyone with insulin dependent diabetes (IDDM) or for people who have non-insulin dependent diabetes (NIDDM), but now require insulin to control their blood glucose levels.

So, what is a carbohydrate exchange? This is a way of counting how much carbohydrate is eaten in each meal or snack. It is commonly accepted that an exchange is equal to 15 g of carbohydrate. This amount was chosen because it translates into easy-to-remember food quantities:

15 g carbohydrate = 1 exchange of bread = 1 slice of bread
= 1 exchange of fruit = 1 piece of fruit
= 1 exchange of rice = ½ cup of rice

Most carbohydrate foods have been analysed for the carbohydrate content so we can calculate how much of a particular food is an exchange. Lists of carbohydrate exchanges can be obtained from a dietitian. The Royal North Shore Hospital in Sydney also sells a book called *The Traffic Light Guide to Food* which includes a comprehensive carbohydrate exchange list. This can be purchased directly from the Royal North Shore Hospital, diabetes centres and from Diabetes Australia.

The majority of carbohydrates exchanges also contain the same energy content, i.e. each carbohydrate exchange provides approximately 340 kJ (80 kCal).

Your dietitian may have calculated a carbohydrate exchange meal plan for you to help you control the amount of food you eat during the day and how this amount should be spread between meals and snacks. The benefit of the carbohydrate exchange meal plan is that it is a way of increasing the variety in your meals without the worry of greatly disturbing your blood glucose levels. If you usually have two pieces of toast for breakfast, but one day feel like a change, you can safely substitute a piece of fruit and an exchange of diet yoghurt instead and know that your blood glucose levels will be similar. Also, the energy or kilojoule content of your breakfast will be similar and so your weight control diet will not be compromised.

Some people find it difficult to change to the regular eating habits which are important with diabetes. A meal plan showing appropriate quantities of food at meals and snacks can be useful in developing better eating habits.

For people requiring insulin at each meal, the exchange system is a useful starting point in determining how to adjust insulin doses. If a meal contains different amounts of carbohydrate, e.g. when going out for dinner, the carbohydrate content of the meal could be much greater than normal. In this situation, a person familiar with the exchange system could tell with confidence how much extra insulin they may need for that meal.

One downside of using a carbohydrate exchange meal plan is the assumption that all carbohydrate foods are digested at the same rate. Consequently, one assumes that two meals containing the same amount of carbohydrate, but from different foods, will have the same effect on blood glucose levels. As explained, not all carbohydrate foods are digested at the same rate and this may cause variations in blood glucose levels. Usually these variations are not enormous, but some people find it useful to use more slowly digested foods to help control their blood glucose levels after meals.

Another criticism of this system is that it may suggest that because the carbohydrate is 'counted', the amount must be limited. This is not the aim of the system; it is simply a way to quantify the amount of carbohydrate eaten, not necessarily limit its content in the diet.

Some people find the lists of carbohydrate exchanges quite daunting and therefore find the system too cumbersome to use.

Please discuss any of these difficulties with your dietitian so they can be clarified. Bear in mind that meal plans are individualised and should be updated regularly, particularly in children and adolescents. The carbohydrate exchange per meal and snack will need to be increased to enable adequate growth and development in children, as well as satisfying their appetite.

ARTIFICIAL SWEETENERS

This area has caused some controversy over the years. Do artificial sweeteners cause cancer? Are they necessary? Should people with diabetes just get used to having fewer sweet foods?

The scientific evidence regarding their possible cancer-causing effects is quite extensive and the artificial sweeteners currently on the market in Australia do not increase the risk of developing cancer. Nutrition scientists would agree that it is better to have a variety of artificial sweeteners available for use so that we do not get an overload of any one particular type of sweetener.

The artificial sweetening agents registered for use in Australia are:
- aspartame (Nutrasweet)
- cyclamate
- saccharine
- sucralose (Splenda)
- acesulphame potassium (Sunnet)
- isomalt
- polydextrose

Note

The sweeteners suitable for use in pregnancy are: aspartame (Nutrasweet), sucralose (Splenda), and acesulphame potassium (Sunnet). This is because they do not cross into the placenta and therefore cannot enter the baby's bloodstream.

All these artificial sweeteners have no nutritional value. In other words, they contain no energy (kilojoules), vitamins, minerals etc. Consequently, they are called *non-nutritive sweeteners*. However, there are other sweetening agents which are sometimes used by the food industry which do have a substantial energy value. These sweeteners will be digested by the body in the same way as sugar and will also lead to a rise in blood glucose levels. We call them *nutritive sweeteners* and they are best avoided — i.e. sorbitol, mannitol, xylitol and fructose.

These sweetening agents can often be identified by the claim on the packaging saying 'carbohydrate modified'. With an increasing range of non-nutritive sweeteners on the market, the place for these other sweeteners is rapidly disappearing. Once again, keep reading the food labels when shopping and, if you find these inappropriate sweeteners in the ingredient list, choose another.

Whether or not you decide to use artificial sweeteners is a personal decision, as seen in the following examples:

> Mrs T did not have a 'sweet tooth', although she did enjoy the occasional spread of jam or honey on her toast and $^1/_2$ teaspoon of sugar in her tea. After diagnosis of her diabetes, Mrs T tried several artificial sweeteners and sugar-free jams, but didn't really enjoy the taste. After discussion with her dietitian, she went back to her previous level of sugar consumption. Her blood glucose levels remained in the normal range and she still lost weight.

> Mr L just loved his fizzy drinks, he drank three cans a day. As well as that, he used three teaspoons of sugar in each of his eight cups of coffee a day. Mr L's dietitian suggested that by replacing the sugar in his drinks with artificial sweetener, he could save 4176 kJ (994 kCal) a day. With that saving, he was free to indulge in a small piece of cake a couple of times a week. The new taste took a bit of getting used to, but seeing that weight loss gave him all the motivation he needed to stick with it. Now he wouldn't drink anything else.

WHAT ABOUT FIBRE?

Fibre is the indigestible part of food which comes from plant sources. Animal foods do not contain any fibre.

Fibre in a diet helps regulate bowel movements and may also help regulate blood glucose levels and help reduce cholesterol. A diet rich in fibre is also encouraged to reduce the risk of some types of cancer. Fibre is certainly filling and can be an invaluable way to help reduce the hunger pangs associated with dietary adjustments.

Experts have agreed that an adult should aim for a daily fibre intake of 30 g. For children, 5 g fibre plus the age of the child is recommended each day, e.g. a child aged 4 years needs 9 g fibre per day. Food labels will show the fibre content of food.

For further information, consult the booklet *Fat and Fibre Counter* by Rosemary Stanton.

WHAT ABOUT CHOLESTEROL AND TRIGLYCERIDES?

Cholesterol is a type of fat made in the body and it has many essential functions. Unfortunately, when the level of cholesterol in the blood gets too high, it is deposited on the walls of the blood vessels. This build-up of cholesterol can restrict blood flow, preventing the tissues from receiving an adequate supply of oxygen and nutrients. In extreme situations, this can cause a heart attack or stroke.

Cholesterol is made from the fat in food. Saturated fats (mainly animal fats) are the biggest culprit. The cholesterol already found in food, such as in eggs and prawns, contributes less to the blood's cholesterol level than the fat eaten.

The dietary advice to lower cholesterol is the same as that found in the dietary guidelines on page 26, i.e. low in fat and high in fibre. Sometimes dietary treatment alone is not enough to bring the cholesterol down to normal and drugs are prescribed to help. The tablets do not replace the use of a healthy, low-fat diet to treat high cholesterol, but are used in conjunction with dietary measures.

Triglycerides are another type of fat found in the blood. They can sometimes be found in high levels by themselves, or in conjunction with high cholesterol. Triglycerides are increased with increased sugar and alcohol in the diet. Poorly controlled diabetes and obesity can also contribute to high triglyceride levels. Weight loss, exercise and improved diabetes control can be useful in lowering the levels.

COOKING FOR HEALTH

Now the lean meats have been selected and the low-fat dairy foods purchased, are there any cooking methods to be aware of which help with the low-fat eating plan? The answer is yes. Below are a selection of cooking ideas to help keep the low-fat food low in fat.
- The most suitable cooking methods are those that require no or minimal fat to be added: i.e. grilling, poaching, boiling, steaming, barbecuing, microwaving or roasting on a rack.

- If frying, use a nonstick pan or a little spray oil to stop the food from sticking. Discard all fat which comes out of the food.
- To grill successfully, place the meat under a hot grill, the meat will cook quickly and not dry out.
- When baking, put the joint of meat or chicken on a rack in a baking tray. Pour 1/2 cup of water into the tray. This will provide moisture during cooking and help prevent the meat from drying out.
- To bake potatoes, brush oil over them using a pastry brush rather than sitting them in a bath of oil. Always use monounsaturated or polyunsaturated cooking oil, e.g. olive oil, canola oil, sunflower oil, corn oil, etc.
- Extend casseroles and mince dishes by substituting a 1/4 of the meat with dried beans, e.g. red kidney beans, butter beans, baked beans etc.
- If you are looking for more low-fat hot breakfast ideas, try baked beans or spaghetti on toast. Grilled mushrooms, with or without tomatoes as a topping, and asparagus spears on toast are other good ideas.
- Low-fat plain yoghurt can be used as a substitute for sour cream in baked potatoes, dips and casseroles. Mix with puréed fruit for a dessert topping.
- Buttermilk can be used as a salad dressing when mixed with lemon juice, herbs, low-joule salad dressing or a small quantity of low-fat mayonnaise. It can also be used instead of margarine in mashed potatoes or in place of sour cream in casseroles.
- Cottage and ricotta cheese can both be used as a dip with corn relish, grated vegetables or curry powder. Serve with vegetable sticks. They can also be used inside baked potatoes or as a substitute for cream cheese. In this case, blend cottage and ricotta cheese in equal proportions.
- Skim fat from casseroles and soups after cooking.
- Stir-fry in a wok or pan with small amounts of aromatic oils, e.g. sesame or olive oil. Use stock, soy sauce and/or sherry to give extra liquid.

- Be adventurous with the use of herbs and spices to add interesting flavour to low-fat meals.
- Marinating meat and poultry helps to keep them tender and add extra flavour. Use any combination of spices, herbs, garlic, lemon rind/juice, mustard, wine.
- Use low-fat milk to make custard, rice pudding, junket, milk jelly etc.

Chapter 7

Exercise

Exercise is something some people love, others hate and some do not give a thought to. Whatever the approach, most people do not do enough exercise. Every day, people are encouraged to do more — of different types, of greater length or of higher intensity — but mainly, just to start exercising. This chapter describes the benefits of doing some exercise and gives practical advice on doing it successfully.

For most people, the idea of exercise conjures up frightening images of Lycra, loud music and the need to look the part before even entering the local gym. These images usually produce more sweat than if the person actually participated in any exercise at all. However, exercise has little to do with gyms and coloured Lycra. It's to do with activity of the body, which involves the actions of various muscles and the lungs. For some, this can be simply walking around the block or doing yoga; for others, it is going for a 10-km jog in the park or a 1-km swim in the pool. Exercise types vary, as does the duration and the intensity. It depends on people's fitness, health and needs. No matter which way it is looked at, there is a type of exercise for everyone. There is a definite health benefit from being more active in daily life, even if the increase of activity is small.

GENERAL BENEFITS OF EXERCISE

Exercise can improve general health and in the long run, decrease the risks of long-term diabetic complications. The general benefits of exercise are substantial. Regular exercise:
- provides the body with more energy, i.e. it makes the muscles work more efficiently;

- strengthens the heart — the heart is a muscle and it can get stronger through exercise;
- improves the circulation — it improves the blood flow around the body, which is especially important in the legs and feet;
- strengthens all muscles — these are what keep us moving so they need to be strong to cope with the pounding they are going to get over the years;
- helps with flexibility — the more flexible the body, the more it can cope with the jarring it is going to get, therefore reducing the risk of injury;
- particularly aerobic exercise, improves breathing, i.e. fitness;
- helps manage weight — either weight loss or maintenance of weight;
- improves blood pressure — it can lower the blood pressure, which can help protect eyes, kidneys and the heart;
- lowers the levels of harmful blood fats — LDL (bad) cholesterol and triglycerides — which can clog the arteries and damage the heart;
- increases HDL (good) cholesterol, which protects large blood vessels and the heart; and
- reduces stress as it helps to release endorphins or 'happy' hormones, which make people feel good.

THE EFFECTS OF EXERCISE IN DIABETES

In addition to these general benefits, regular exercise improves overall blood glucose control for people with diabetes, especially people with non-insulin dependent diabetes (NIDDM).

Exercise involves the use of muscles and these require a fuel supply to work. This fuel is glucose, and a steady supply of it is required when exercising, mainly from the food that is eaten. Only a limited supply of glucose can be stored in the muscle itself and it always needs replenishing. This replenishment goes on long after the exercise has finished. The longer the exercise and the higher the intensity, the longer it takes to replenish these stores. This may lead to hypos several hours after the exercise has finished (*see* chapter 11, 'Hypoglycaemia').

Regular exercise in people with NIDDM can lead to an improvement in the sensitivity to insulin. NIDDM is characterised by insulin resistance. Exercise can improve this resistance and make the body more sensitive. The body then needs less insulin to control the blood glucose and may therefore lower the need for medication. People with either insulin dependent diabetes (IDDM) or NIDDM may find that, with regular exercise, they require less insulin or tablets to control their blood glucose levels.

In people with IDDM, exercise improves overall fitness, reduces the risk of cardiovascular problems and improves the body's overall response to insulin. Most people who have IDDM from a young age should be encouraged, like everyone else, to get out and enjoy an active life. Sports are good for social development, self-confidence and psychological wellbeing.

GETTING OUT THERE...AND DOING IT

If the benefits of exercise are so extensive and worthwhile, why does the mere thought of exercise often bring on pangs of guilt, despair and sheer terror? Excuses, excuses! Being too tired or too busy to exercise is one of the most common excuses used when people are asked about this topic. Others state they just do not like it, 'My health won't let me', 'My balance is poor and I might fall', 'I'm too old', 'I get bored', 'It's too difficult to get to and I get lonely'. For every excuse used, there is usually a solution. So beware when thinking up an excuse to tell health professionals, they have heard most of them anyway!

The biggest problem is the fact that no one can really make anyone else exercise, short of physically dragging them out of bed to walk around the block. Deep down, a person really has to *decide* to do it and start making changes to their overall lifestyle forever. Overcoming some of the barriers that people feel exist is the first step. Below are some hints that may help:

- Do not overdo it at first; set short-term goals and build up gradually, e.g. tackling a marathon first up may put someone off running for life.
- Find a friend or a dog to participate; having someone else along is great motivation.
- Choose something that is enjoyable and is physically achievable.
- Vary the type of exercise or change the route after a while to keep up your interest.
- Try and incorporate exercise into your daily life, e.g. walk to or from work, get off a few stops earlier from the train or bus and walk the rest of the way or use the stairs instead of lifts.

- Get up a little earlier to exercise or, in summer, do it in the evenings while it is still light.

HOW MUCH EXERCISE IS NECESSARY?

In order to gain real health benefits, such as cardiovascular fitness, diabetes control and weight loss or weight maintenance, you need to do the following:

- Exercise for 30–45 minutes, three to five times a week. Exercise needs to be done at a moderately active rate in order to gain the best glucose- and fat-burning effects for the body. Of course, this is not possible for everyone, but anything less than three times a week will not provide the major long-term benefits. However, something is always better than nothing, and increasing exercise over several months may increase the amount achieved substantially.
- The intensity of exercise varies amongst individuals due to age, physical fitness and medical conditions. These factors all play a part in determining how much exercise a person can manage. Feeling slightly puffed at the end of the session, but still able to talk, is a good way to determine if the exercise has been beneficial. Of course, overdoing it and ending up with a red face and suffering exhaustion is not a good idea unless this is your regular exercise routine and you are medically fit to carry it out.
- Build up the exercise routine and the intensity gradually over weeks or months.

TYPES AND TAPES

Aerobic forms of exercise are the best as they require the use of oxygen to burn the fuel in the muscle. Being aerobically fit enables the body to work more efficiently and improve heart, lungs, blood vessels, weight and blood glucose control. Exercises such as walking, swimming, cycling and jogging are good examples as they require energy to burn which would normally be stored as fat. This is great for weight loss. There are many other types of aerobic exercises, e.g. dancing, surfing, skiing, tennis, tai chi, aerobics and cycling.

The other type of exercise is anaerobic exercise. Anaerobic exercise does not require the use of oxygen. For instance, weightlifting develops muscular strength and endurance. Used alone, it will not benefit blood glucose control or weight loss. Used in conjunction with aerobic exercise, however, it will provide better tone and strength to the aerobically fit body.

Deciding to exercise is hard enough, but finding out about the choices available around your local area can be even more of a challenge. If exercising in isolation is not your thing, look around for local councils, sporting clubs and senior citizens or community health centres, which usually run some form of exercise groups or at least have information about what is available. There is also a variety of exercise videos on the market. Even the fashion top models are making some, showing everyone how easy it is too look like them (don't we wish). For people with mobility problems, there are good armchair exercise tapes available. Try the local library or health centres.

PRACTICAL ASPECTS FOR PEOPLE WITH DIABETES WHO TAKE TABLETS OR INSULIN

Monitoring

Exercise makes the blood glucose drop by increasing the rate at which muscles take up glucose. Therefore, make sure to take a blood glucose level before exercise, after it finishes and later on, to ensure that the glucose level is not too low, especially before going to bed. If the exercise is going to be intense and last a long time, it is a good idea to test during exercise as well. Note that exercise improved the body's response to insulin for up to 15 hours (sometimes even longer), so watch out for a low blood glucose level for up to 15 hours after vigorous exercise.

If the test prior to exercise is above 15mmol/L it is best not to exercise. A high blood glucose level indicates a lack of circulating insulin and the body may instead produce more glucose from the liver during exercise and actually make the glucose level rise. In people with IDDM, this may also produce ketones and drive the glucose even higher, leading to diabetic ketoacidosis (*see* chapter 12, 'The highs of diabetes').

Adjustment of carbohydrate and/or insulin

It is necessary to adjust intake of carbohydrate and/or insulin when exercising, particularly if the exercise is going to be strenuous and prolonged. Everybody has different insulin requirements, but usually a reduction of perhaps 10% or more in the doses of insulin working at the time of exercise and for 10–15 hours afterwards is desirable. This can be discussed with your doctor or diabetes educator. Some carbohydrate can be eaten before and/or during the exercise. Discuss appropriate food choices with a dietitian. Performing blood glucose monitoring will also help to determine how much carbohydrate is required before and during exercise. Always remember to carry some quick-acting glucose with you such as jelly beans, sugar cubes or glucose tablets. Do not inject insulin into an area that is going to be exercised as this will cause faster absorption and action of the insulin. Use the abdomen, unless the exercise planned is going to be sit-ups. If a person is overweight, it is best to reduce insulin or tablets rather than to increase carbohydrate intake to avoid hypoglycaemia.

General considerations

1. Prior to commencement of an exercise program, people more than 35 years who have had diabetes for more than 10 years need to have a check-up with a doctor to make sure the heart, lungs and eyes are in good order (especially if no exercise has been done before). The exercise routine has to be suitable for your body's ability and fitness level. If you do get unduly short of breath or have pain in the chest when exercising, stop and report immediately to your doctor.
2. Examine your feet before taking that big step out the door and upon return. Look for blisters, cuts or potential problem areas such as red spots or corns that could lead to a blister forming. Make sure that shoes fit well, are of good quality, are supportive and are not brand new.
3. People treated with medication should always carry simple sugar such as jelly beans or glucose tablets to eat in case of hypoglycaemia while exercising.
4. Drink plenty of water to keep well hydrated.
5. Warm up and cool down for a short period before and after exercise to avoid soft tissue damage.

6. Exercise in the cooler part of the day in summer and in winter when it is warmer, and always dress appropriately.

People have very different goals for exercising. Goals should be realistic and need to be reviewed and/or modified so there is always a sense of achievement. Remember the long-term benefits do outweigh the temporary excuses not to exercise. It all comes down to a positive attitude and careful planning, with support from a health team.

Chapter 8

Insulin Delivery

When people with diabetes require insulin, various models of delivering the insulin are available, e.g. syringes, pens and pumps. Syringes and insulin pens are the most commonly used modes of delivery.

SYRINGES

Currently in Australia, insulin syringes come in four sizes: 0.25 mL, 0.3 mL, 0.5 mL and 1.0 mL. The measurement markings or gradations on the side of the syringe vary according to the size of the syringe.

The 0.5 mL syringe

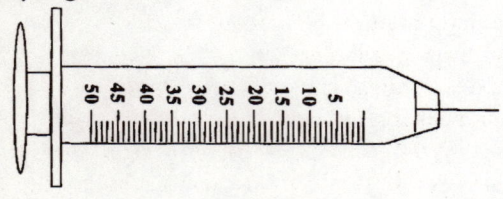

As shown in the diagram each line or gradation on the 0.5 mL syringe equals 1 unit of insulin.

The 1.0 mL syringe

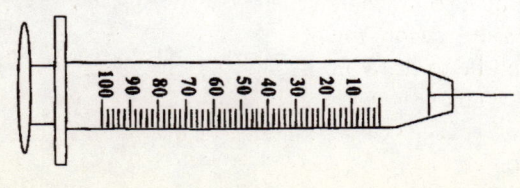

As demonstrated in the diagram, each line or gradation on the 1.0 mL syringe equals 2 units of insulin. Numbers appearing on the syringe increase by increments of ten, e.g. 10, 20, 30 up to 100 units.

The needles for the end of the syringe come in varying thicknesses and lengths. The thickness of the needle is referred to as the 'gauge'. Needles are available in 27-, 29- and 30-gauge. The 30-gauge is the finest needle available for insulin syringes. The needles are available in various lengths, these being 8 mm, 12 mm and 12.7 mm.

INSULIN PENS

Administering insulin via an insulin pen has become very popular. The insulin is stored in a cartridge inside the pen and the number of units is 'dialled up', then the dose given as with a syringe and vial. This makes things much easier when in public or in a social setting. The attachable needles for insulin pens are available in varied sizes. Needles for insulin pens are available in 28, 29, and 30 and 31 gauge; 31 gauge being the finest size. Needles for insulin pens are available in 8-mm and 12-mm lengths.

When using an insulin pen, people are advised to leave the needle in the injected site for a few seconds after injecting the insulin to ensure complete delivery of the required insulin dose. Follow the manufacturer's instructions when using an insulin pen.

Cartridges are available with quick-acting, intermediate-acting and pre-mixed insulins. However, there are some disadvantages to using insulin pens instead of syringes, for example it is not possible to mix two different insulins in the same pen, as can be done with a syringe. To give both an intermediate-acting and a quick-acting insulin at the same time would require two separate pens and two separate injections, unless the pen is loaded with a pre-mixed insulin. Therefore, it is common for people to use a syringe and vial at home for intermediate-acting insulin, and an insulin pen for their quick-acting insulin when they are away from home during the day.

If, for some reason, the pen breaks down, the only way of giving insulin will be to draw up insulin directly from the cartridge with a syringe. Thus, it is very important that every patient knows how to draw up with a syringe, even if they normally use a pen. (Having a back-up pen is a good idea.) Imagine if you were stuck in a lift overnight or on a delayed flight with a broken pen, and with a syringe as a back-up. Pens have certainly made the business of giving insulin a lot easier for many people, but as with everything there are pros and cons to be considered.

PUMPS

Sometimes people who have had extreme difficulty in controlling their blood glucose levels with the usual insulin injections use insulin pumps to give insulin in a manner more like that of the pancreas. The pump (about cigarette-pack size) is connected to a subcutaneous (under the skin) needle. The pump rate can be adjusted so that insulin is pumped in quickly during meals, but at a slower rate in between meals.

Frequent blood glucose testing is essential to decide on rate changes and disconnecting the pump for any length of time can lead to ketoacidosis. Pumps are expensive and involve more time and trouble than injections. They also have other disadvantages, such as local infections where the needle enters the skin. For most people, a pump is more troublesome and no better than multiple injections using a pen. However, a small number of people with very 'brittle' diabetes seem to gain extra benefit from using a pump.

INJECTION SITE

Insulin can be injected into one of a number of different sites, e.g. the abdomen, upper arms, thighs or buttocks. The abdomen is the most ideal site to use. Absorption of insulin is considered to be most consistent from the abdomen. When preparing and giving insulin by syringe the following diagramatic instructions included in this chapter may be useful to follow.

It is strongly recommended that the site of injection be rotated within the abdominal area, and a different injection site chosen each time. If you keep injecting in the same spot, a fatty lump will develop (fat hypertrophy) and the absorption of insulin into the bloodstream will be more erratic.

INSULIN ALLERGIES

Ever since insulin injections have been used, there have been some people who had an allergic response to the injections. This was more common when insulin was prepared from animals and not as purified as it is now. The insulin currently in use is mostly identical to human insulin and has virtually no other contaminants. Rarely, people are allergic to the solutions in which the insulins come. Occasionally, there is a genuine allergy to the insulin molecule itself. Whatever the cause, very little insulin allergy occurs nowadays.

Someone with an allergy, at first usually feels itchy around the site of injection. There may also be generalised body itching, weals and some swelling. Very rarely, the allergy can cause wheezing and breathing difficulty. The sufferer can be tested to reveal what the allergy is due to and, if necessary, a desensitisation treatment can be given.

LIPOATROPHY OR LIPOHYPERTROPHY

When the insulins injected were less pure, it was not uncommon to see some excess growth of the fat tissue in the injection areas (lipohypertrophy), usually the thighs. Less commonly, there was thinning of these fatty areas (lipoatrophy). This resulted in an unsatisfactory cosmetic appearance and could also make the absorption of insulin unreliable, depending on the lumpiness of the area into which it was injected.

Today, with pure insulins, these changes are much less common. Rotating the injection sites will help prevent the lumpiness caused by injecting into the same place. Occasionally, liposuction may be needed to remove the lumpiness.

STORAGE OF INSULIN

Insulin can be stored for a period of time until the expiry period has been reached. Do not use insulin which is past the expiry date written on the bottle.

The most effective way to store insulin is laying it on its side in the refrigerator, which should be between 2°C and 8°C. Do not freeze insulin. The bottle of insulin in use can be kept out of the refrigerator, but must not be exposed to extreme temperatures, e.g. do not leave it on the dashboard or in the glove box of the car. Insulin stored out of the refrigerator should be discarded after 1 month.

Drawing up insulin

1. Mix the insulin by rolling the bottle between hands.

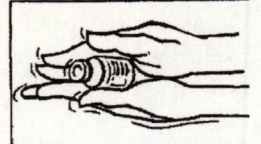

2. Pull down the syringe handle until the top black line moves to the correct number of units marked on the syringe barrel.

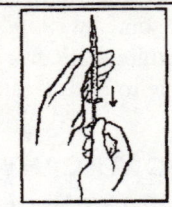

3. Push needle through the rubber bottle seal. Push down handle all the way.

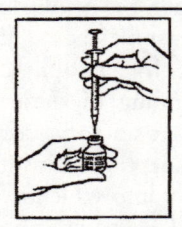

4. With needle still in the bottle turn both upside down. Pull down handle until the top black line moves to the correct number of units marked on the syringe barrel.

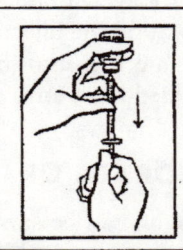

5. Hold syringe by the barrel and pull the needle out of the bottle.

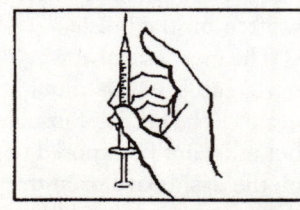

Mixing Insulin

1. Roll and mix **'cloudy'** insulin.

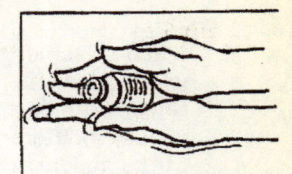

2. Inject air into **'cloudy'**.

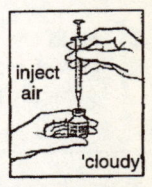

3. Inject air into **'clear'**.

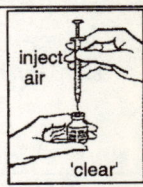

4. Draw up dose of **'clear'** insulin.

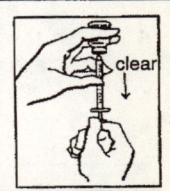

5. Draw up dose of **'cloudy'** insulin. Do not squirt any excess insulin back into vial.

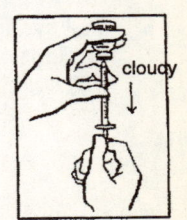

Giving an insulin injection

1. Pinch up some fat on your abdomen.
   Note: With each injection choose a different part of the abdomen to inject.

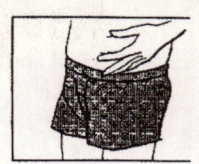

2. Hold the syringe by its barrel, like a dart pointing straight at the skin.

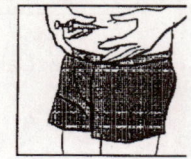

3. Push needle through the skin. Push it in all the way.

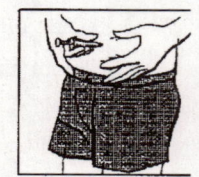

4. Push the handle down all the way.

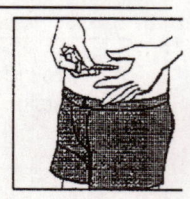

5. Pull syringe and needle straight out of the skin.

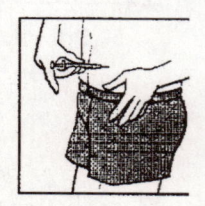

The Diabetes Centre, St. Vincent's Hospital, Sydney

Chapter 9

Insulin Therapy in IDDM

In this chapter, the types and actions of insulin currently in use are described. Devices for giving insulin are also described and some basic information on adjusting insulin dosages is given.

Our bodies normally require insulin to be present at all times (even if in very small amounts), in order to keep blood glucose levels normal. Insulin is also necessary to prevent breakdown of fat, which can lead to build-up of acids in the blood (ketoacidosis). Thus, the pancreas usually produces some insulin 24 hours a day, and releases extra insulin in response to meals.

In insulin dependent diabetes mellitus (IDDM), the pancreas produces little or no insulin at all. Therefore, the insulin needs to be replaced by injections, as insulin is not absorbed whole when taken by mouth. For these reasons, it is important that there is insulin in the body 24 hours a day: this is the most important priority.

With injected insulin, it is best to mimic the normal action of the pancreas in releasing more insulin at meal times. For people with IDDM, this requires at least two injections, and more usually three or four. Some people with non-insulin dependent diabetes (NIDDM) will eventually require insulin treatment. However, this usually will be only one or two injections per day as there will be some insulin being made in the pancreas.

TYPES OF INSULIN PREPARATIONS

The different insulin preparations all contain the same insulin. What is different is that with which the insulin is mixed. Different mixtures are used to slow down the rate at which the insulin is absorbed from under the skin and into the bloodstream. In this way, only one or two injections per day can provide a '24-hour' supply of insulin. The quicker acting preparations can be used to provide a 'burst' of insulin around meal times.

There are insulin preparations that are released sufficiently slowly so that a single injection can provide a 24-hour supply (Ultratard, Humulin UL). However, it is usually more reliable to give an intermediate-acting insulin (Protaphane, Humulin NPH, Monotard) twice a day, or once a day in combination with a quick-acting insulin (Actrapid, Humulin R and Humalog) before meals.

The action profiles of the various insulin preparations (i.e. the rate at which they are absorbed from under the skin and released into your 'system') can be displayed in pictorial form. It should be stressed, however, that these profiles represent averages, and the differences between people and even within the same person on different days can be quite large, so that they are a rough guide only.

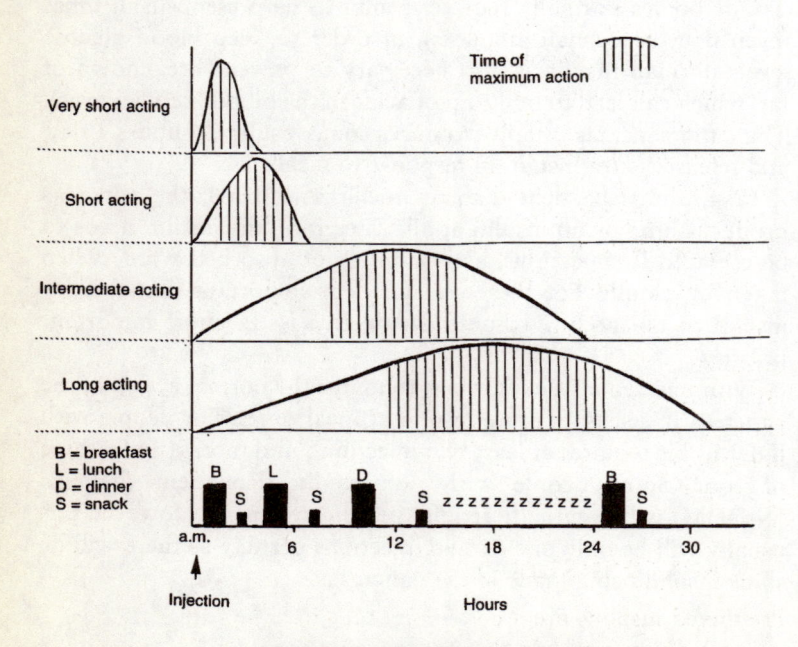

TIME - ACTION OF VARIOUS INSULINS

Sample insulin regimens include:
- ONCE-DAILY INJECTION OF LONG-ACTING INSULIN. There are major drawbacks with the single injection approach – day-to-day variation in the action profile may mean periods of no insulin in the body with consequent risk of high blood glucose and ketoacidosis. Also, any adjustments to amounts of insulin can only be made once per day and it is not really possible to make fine adjustments to the daily blood glucose patterns.
- TWICE-DAILY INJECTION OF INTERMEDIATE-ACTING INSULIN. This gives a more reliable 24-hour cover than the once-daily injection outlined above. There are now two times in the day that adjustments can be made, allowing doses to be tailored more closely to day-to-day requirements. Quite satisfactory control can often be achieved on this type of regimen, particularly if the person can manage to have a fairly routine lifestyle, i.e. no major day-to-day variations in amount and timing of food and activities.
- EVENING DOSE OF INTERMEDIATE-ACTING INSULIN WITH QUICK-ACTING INSULIN BEFORE EACH MEAL. This is known as a 'basal bolus' regimen and can involve four injections per day. The evening injection provides insulin overnight and daytime requirements are provided by the quick-acting insulin. The frequency of injection allows short-term adjustments to be made to allow for variations in meal time, meal size and exercise levels. It is most suited to the busy, active person and will not be suitable or necessary for everyone.

There are numerous variations and combinations of the above regimens and no single type will suit everybody. Sometimes intermediate-acting insulin is given twice daily along with quick-acting injections; quick-acting may be given before some meals and not others etc. It is a matter of finding the best combination for the individual concerned.

PRE-MIXED INSULINS

Pre-mixed insulins are a combination of intermediate- and quick-acting insulin mixed in the same container. The most popular is '30/70', which is 30% quick acting and 70% intermediate acting. Also available are '50/50' and '20/80'. Pre-mixed insulins are useful because, in the case of syringes and vials, the insulins do not need to be mixed daily in the syringe or, in the case of pens (see page 59), mixing insulin does not require two separate injections. However, the disadvantage is that the proportions of the quick-and intermediate-acting insulins cannot be adjusted independently, thus reducing flexibility in making dosage adjustments to improve blood glucose control or to prevent hypoglycaemia (see page 81). Pre-mixed insulins may not suit everyone, particularly people with very active, unpredictable lifestyles.

ADJUSTMENT OF INSULIN

The blood glucose level at any moment in time is the result of the balance between three major forces acting at once, namely:
1. insulin;
2. sugar release into the blood either from food eaten or stored in the liver; and
3. exercise.

As sugar release into the blood and exercise can vary widely from minute to minute and hour to hour, it is usually the insulin levels that smooth the blood glucose levels out. In people without diabetes, the amount of insulin being released from the pancreas can be turned up or down very quickly as needed. However, when insulin is injected under the skin it is absorbed and released at a more or less constant rate, regardless of what the blood glucose level is at that time. Thus, the amount and sometimes the timing of insulin injections may have to be adjusted to cope with anticipated variations in food intakes and or exercise. You have to try and pretend to be a pancreas!

Frequently when people with diabetes find their blood glucose is high, they inject some quick-acting insulin to bring the level down. While sometimes this is a good idea, it is not favoured as a regular way of controlling blood glucose levels. It is looking back rather than forward — treating a level that has already become too high. It is better to ask, 'How can I prevent this happening tomorrow?' The answer is by adjusting the amount of insulin in advance next time.

SOME USEFUL POINTS TO FOLLOW

It is usual to give some intermediate-acting insulin in the evening. This provides insulin in the 'system' overnight. As the body prepares to face the new day (even before you have woken up), the 'stress' hormones (*see* chapter 1, 'What is diabetes?') which will raise the blood glucose levels are released if there is not insulin present to counteract them. Having sufficient insulin acting overnight can help prevent this. However, if too much insulin is given in the evening, there is a risk of having a low blood glucose level in the middle of the night without being aware of it (because we do not eat in our sleep). This is less likely to happen if the 'overnight' insulin is given at bedtime (9–10 p.m.) rather than at meal time. If you are also having quick-acting insulin before dinner, it requires 'splitting the dose' and does require an extra injection.

There are a couple of useful ideas to prevent night-time hypoglycaemia:

- Do not go to bed with a blood glucose level less than 7 mmol/L. If it is less than 7 mmol/L, have an extra carbohydrate snack.
- If there is any suspicion of night-time hypoglycaemia, set the alarm clock for around 3 a.m. and check the blood glucose level at this time. You can then adjust the night-time insulin or snack to prevent this from happening in the future.

PROBLEM	ACTION
Blood glucose level on waking low	Reduce evening dose of too intermediate-acting insulin
Blood glucose level on waking too high	Increase evening dose of intermediate-acting insulin (be careful to check that the blood glucose level earlier in the night is not low)

As can be seen, the blood glucose level in the morning is controlled by the insulin given the night before. This is generally the case with intermediate-acting insulin — as shown in the diagram of insulin action on page 66. Intermediate-acting insulins have their main effect on blood glucose levels 'down the track'.

As quick-acting insulins are released a lot more rapidly, they are used to provide a burst of insulin to coincide with meal time, as does the normal pancreas. They take approximately 30 minutes to get into the blood so it is usual to give them about 30 minutes before a meal. A newly available type of insulin called *lispro insulin* (brand name Humalog) is absorbed very quickly (about 5 minutes), allowing insulin to be taken at meal time instead of prior to the meal. This may allow greater flexibility in timing and planning of meals. Through experimentation, the dose required to cope with different size meals can be found. Only give a quick-acting insulin injection if you are in 'sight' of food – do not give it in a lift or on the highway unless you have a back-up snack available. Likewise, it is a 'no-no' to take insulin and skip a scheduled meal deliberately.

Exercise usually reduces blood glucose levels because the muscles 'burn up' the sugar. To do this properly, however, requires the presence of insulin. If there is insufficient insulin present, the blood glucose may actually go up in response to exercise. Thus, if the blood glucose is high to begin with (which may indicate that there is insufficient insulin in the body), the situation may be made worse rather than better by exercise. It is important to understand what exercising in this situation can do (*see* chapter 7, 'Exercise').

Exercise allows insulin to work better, often for up to 15 hours after the exercise has finished, because it has made the muscles more sensitive to insulin. Exercise can lower the blood glucose level for many hours afterwards. Therefore, the insulin doses given some time after vigorous exercise may have to be reduced somewhat.

As can be seen, the interaction between insulin, food and exercise can be very complex, and no two individuals are the same. Everyone will differ in the degree to which changes in these three things affect the blood glucose level. Some examples of how adjustments may be made follow.

PROBLEM	ACTION
Blood glucose level mid-morning too high	Increase quick-acting insulin before breakfast or consider whether breakfast is too large.
Blood glucose level mid-morning too low	Decrease quick-acting insulin before breakfast or consider whether you are skipping breakfast. Also, did you exercise more than usual after breakfast?

The same principles apply to high or low blood glucose levels in the afternoon or after dinner.

Chapter 10

Medication in NIDDM

In earlier chapters, it was emphasised that the cornerstones of diabetic management are an appropriate food intake in combination with regular exercise. Often the blood glucose level will be controlled initially by diet alone. However, after a variable period of time, blood glucose levels may become higher despite an appropriate diet, regular exercise and ideal body weight. If and when this occurs, tablets are usually introduced. At present, there are two main groups of tablets in common usage. These will be discussed in this chapter. Other types of tablets which will soon become available are also described.

People with non-insulin dependent diabetes mellitus (NIDDM) do produce and release insulin, although in reduced amounts. In most people with NIDDM, there is a progressive decline in the amount of insulin produced by the pancreas. Consequently, there is a rise in the blood glucose level necessitating the introduction of tablets to control the diabetes effectively. In time, higher doses of tablets and/or a combination of different tablets are required. Eventually maximum doses of tablets are reached and, with any further rise in blood glucose levels, insulin needs to be used. Insulin can be used alone or it may be used together with one or other type of tablet.

For example:

> Mr D.M. was a 53-year-old man who presented to his local doctor with a generalised feeling of tiredness and lack of energy. On closer questioning, it was discovered that he had gained 7 kg over the past year. He had not noticed any thirst and specifically denied passing more urine than normal. He admitted to drinking three glasses of beer each day (more on

weekends) and, when asked about his diet, it was discovered that he rarely ate breakfast, had one or two meat pies for lunch and had a large evening meal.

It was noted that his mother had developed diabetes in her early 60s, but there was no one else in the family with diabetes. He had been treated for high blood pressure for the past 5 years.

When he was originally seen he weighed 103 kg and was 175 cm tall. A random blood sugar level was 17mmol/L, which confirmed that he had diabetes.

Initially he was seen by a dietitian, encouraged to exercise regularly and taught to test his blood glucose levels. When reviewed one month later, he had changed his diet and was walking regularly for at least half an hour each day. He was testing his blood glucose levels regularly. Most blood sugars were between 5 and 8 mmol/L. Three months later, he had lost 5 kg in weight and blood glucose levels ranged between 4 and 7 mmol/L.

ORAL AGENTS (TABLETS)

Biguanides

Biguanides were first used in 1957 and metformin (trade names: Diabex, Diaformin, Glucophage) is the only currently available member of this group. The mechanism by which metformin lowers the blood glucose level is less clear than for sulphonylureas. Probably their major effect is to increase the sensitivity of both liver and muscle to the action of insulin. Metformin also causes a delay of carbohydrate absorption from the gut and decreases the output of glucose from the liver.

Metformin is a very useful medication, especially in the overweight person with NIDDM. On its own, it is not particularly powerful at lowering the blood sugar. It has its greatest use in the overweight person with a relatively mildly elevated blood glucose level or in combination with either sulphonylureas or insulin.

Example (continued):

Two years later, Mr D.M. had regained 3 kg, but was still 4 kg less than when he was first diagnosed. He was still exercising, although most weeks he would only exercise on three occasions. He tested his blood glucose levels regularly, but values now ranged between 8 and 12 mmol/L. His doctor decided to start treatment with tablets. As he was still significantly overweight, he was started on metformin, which does not cause any weight gain. His starting dose was 500 mg (one tablet) after breakfast.

Mr D.M. started to exercise more regularly, was more strict with his diet and his blood glucose levels improved. Six months later, his blood glucose levels again began to rise and his dose of metformin was increased to one tablet twice a day, after breakfast and after his evening meal.

Metformin is absorbed by the entire gut, is not altered by the body and is excreted by the kidney. Minor gastrointestinal side effects are relatively common and occur in up to 20% of people. These may be transient and are less likely if the initial dose is low and is gradually increased. Gastrointestinal side effects may be less if the metformin is taken after meals. So, if mild symptoms occur, the tablets can be taken after a meal. More severe gastrointestinal upset, including diarrhoea, occurs in a small number of people who cannot continue taking the medication.

An extremely rare complication of treatment with metformin is lactic acidosis. This condition has occurred only in people with kidney, liver or severe cardiovascular disease, or in the very elderly. Therefore, metformin should be avoided or used cautiously in such situations.

SULPHONYLUREAS

Insulin is normally produced and released by beta cells in the pancreas in response to a rise in glucose, i.e. insulin is released as the glucose level in the blood rises. These beta cells are found in islands within the pancreas called islets of Langerhans.

Sulphonylureas are very commonly used in patients with NIDDM who have high blood glucose levels despite their best efforts to control diabetes with a diet and exercise program. There are many different sulphonylureas available with different brand names and each of these is manufactured by a different pharmaceutical company.

The sulphonylurea group of drugs works by stimulating insulin release from the beta cells of the pancreas. More importantly, sulphonylureas improve the release of insulin in response to a rise in blood glucose. Sulphonylureas have other effects, but these are probably minor and without any significant clinical relevance. As they act primarily by causing the release of insulin, they have no effect in anyone who does not secrete insulin.

Sulphonylureas should be taken immediately before eating. Some can be taken once per day and others need to be taken more often – up to three times per day. The various tablets last in the body for a variable period of time depending on the person's kidney and liver functions. They are removed and/or broken down in the body by either the kidney or the liver, or both, so less tablets need to be taken by people with either kidney or liver disease. The dosage of different tablets varies, however, it is usual to start with $1/2$–1 tablet per day and gradually increase the dose until acceptable blood glucose levels are achieved.

Side effects of these tablets are relatively uncommon. The most important side effect is hypoglycaemia (hypo), which can be prolonged and severe. It most often occurs:

1. in the elderly;
2. if there is liver or kidney disease;
3. if a meal has been missed or if the person has had inadequate carbohydrate;
4. if unusual exercise is undertaken;
5. if alcohol has been consumed, especially if inadequate food has been eaten.

The symptoms of hypoglycaemia are described in chapter 11, but may not be typical in the elderly. Anyone who is taking sulphonylureas should be aware of the possibility of hypoglycaemia and how to deal with it.

Other side effects occur rarely. Occasionally, skin rashes, nausea, vomiting or diarrhoea may be experienced. Sulphonylureas should not be used during pregnancy as they may harm the baby. It is also recommended that breastfeeding women do not take sulphonylureas.

Example (continued):

> Some 18 months later, Mr D.M.'s blood glucose levels once again began to rise, despite a continuing diet, regular exercise and increasing doses of

metformin. It was decided to add another type of tablet — the sulphonylureas. Mr D.M. had no kidney or liver problems, so a tablet was chosen which needed to be taken only once or twice a day. Initially, he was started on half a tablet a day, but it was explained that if blood glucose levels remained higher than acceptable, the dose may need to be increased. As time progressed, the sulphonylurea dosage was gradually increased in an effort to control blood glucose levels.

INSULIN

With the passage of time and despite the best efforts of doctors and the person with diabetes, there is often a gradual increase in the tablets required to control blood glucose levels. Eventually, maximum amounts of sulphonylureas and metformin are being taken, but blood glucose levels still remain too high.

At this point, it is important to review the aims of management in diabetes:
1. to preserve quality of life and sense of wellbeing;
2. to prevent diabetic complications; and
3. to avoid hypoglycaemia.

The average time from the diagnosis of diabetes to the necessity for insulin is 8 to 10 years. Of course, sometimes insulin is needed much earlier than this and at other times it may not be required until many years later than the average.

Once people reach the stage of taking the maximum amount of tablets, they are often very reluctant and even frightened to consider insulin. Many relatives and even medical attendants mistakenly believe that they are doing their patient or relative a favour by avoiding insulin. Nothing could be further from the truth. Insulin treatment has advanced so much in recent years that there is very little to fear and there are very few patients who are unable to manage their own insulin treatment.

Example (continued):

> Ten years after the diagnosis of diabetes was made, Mr D.M. was taking maximum doses of both metformin and sulphonylureas. His weight had been stable for some years and he was exercising regularly.

He was testing his blood glucose level every day at different times during the day. Levels before breakfast were ranging between 9 and 12 mmol/L. At other times during the day, blood glucose levels rose as high as 17 mmol/L.

He denied excessive thirst or passing lots of urine, but did admit to a general feeling of tiredness and lack of energy. He was quite reluctant to start insulin, but, after a further month's trial during which his blood glucose levels did not improve, he agreed with some reservation.

It was explained that he would not need to be admitted to hospital and that he would be started on insulin as an outpatient. He was referred to a diabetes centre and started to take an isophane (Protaphane, Humulin NPH) insulin before breakfast and before his evening meal. The diabetes educators showed him what to do. He kept in touch with the diabetes centre by telephone or by dropping in for a short time.

Two weeks later, he was quite comfortable with injecting insulin with a syringe and was stable on a set amount of insulin. Moreover, he had regained his energy and was feeling generally much better. He knew how to plan his exercise and what to do if he had a sick day. It was suggested that, in the future, if he wished, he could learn to use an insulin pen device. His blood glucose levels had improved and most were now once again under 10 mmol/L. He had unfortunately gained 3 kg in weight.

Once blood glucose levels are consistently over 10mmol/L, there is an increased risk of developing diabetic complications such as eye damage (retinopathy), nerve damage (neuropathy) and kidney damage (nephropathy). In addition, the body's defence against infection is impaired. The classical symptoms of diabetes such as thirst and the passage of large quantities of urine are often not present at this time, but not infrequently there is a general feeling of tiredness, lack of energy and a reduced feeling of wellbeing. Once insulin treatment is initiated, most patients notice a vast improvement in the way they feel and very few wish to return to treatment with tablets.

The methods of insulin administration have been covered in earlier chapters but suffice it to say, modern insulin therapy is vastly easier than in years gone by. Today, disposable plastic syringes with very fine needles that have a special lubricant are available, so that the injection under the skin is barely felt. In fact, most people agree that an insulin injection hurts far less than the pinprick required for blood glucose level tests. In addition, pen devices are available which are simple to use and very convenient when you are away from home.

Most people are quite ignorant about modern insulin administration, which is one of the reasons for their fear and reluctance to start treatment. Until 15 years ago, patients were usually admitted to hospital to start insulin. Nowadays this is rarely necessary. With the help of a specialist diabetes nurse educator, virtually everyone can be stabilised on insulin as an outpatient.

Insulin treatment in people with NIDDM is a little different than for those with insulin dependent diabetes mellitus (IDDM). First, people with NIDDM are older; secondly, they are still making and releasing some of their own insulin; and, lastly, very tight control of blood glucose levels may not be absolutely necessary nor even desirable.

The type of insulin, the number of injections per day, the method of administration and the dose of insulin will usually be established at the time of initial stabilisation. The insulin regimen may, of course, be changed from time to time if one of the goals is not being satisfactorily achieved.

Three types of insulin are commonly used by people with NIDDM who require it:

1. quick-acting insulin (Actrapid, Humulin R);
2. intermediate-acting insulin (Protaphane, Humulin NPH, Monotard, Lente); and
3. longer-acting insulin (Ultralente).

In addition, a number of pre-mixed combinations are available. At present, there are pre-mixed insulins with ratios of quick-acting/intermediate-acting insulin of 20%:80%, 30%:70% and 50%:50%.

In Australia, most of the insulin preparations in use are human insulin, but beef isophane insulin (Isotard) is readily available and has a longer duration of action than human isophane. Beef isophane is sometimes used to increase the chance of controlling the diabetes on one injection a day.

As people with NIDDM have some capacity for insulin secretion, their blood glucose levels can often be controlled with twice-daily doses of intermediate-acting insulin without the need for shorter acting insulin. Sometimes they do require the addition of a quick-acting insulin before breakfast and before the evening meal. This can usually be achieved by changing to one of the pre-mixed combinations. Most people do not require more than two injections of insulin per day, although there are exceptions.

In the very elderly, the goals of management are centred on management of symptoms and avoidance of hypoglycaemia rather than on the prevention of future diabetic complications. In these people, and in some cases in younger people, one can often obtain acceptable control with a combination of insulin and sulphonylurea tablets. The insulin may be given either in the morning before breakfast, before the evening meal or at around 10 p.m. Doses and timing of insulin are adjusted according to blood glucose levels performed at home. Sometimes it is easier for people to start insulin therapy this way, by adding a night-time insulin injection to the daily tablets.

Occasionally, metformin is prescribed in combination with insulin. This is particularly useful in the overweight or in someone who requires very large doses of insulin. This is because metformin makes the body more sensitive to insulin whether that insulin is produced by the person or administered via a syringe (or pen device). If the blood glucose control is not adequate when taking tablets and insulin, it usually is best to cease the tablets and take the insulin twice daily.

One of the inevitable consequences of insulin therapy is weight gain. Most studies have shown that between 2 and 4 kg of weight is gained, although one recent study demonstrated an average 10-kg weight gain! Some weight gain is largely unavoidable, but it can be limited by an appropriate exercise program and diet, and sometimes by use of metformin with the insulin. Some weight is regained because the improvement in blood glucose levels prevents continuing loss of glucose in the urine.

NEWER MEDICATIONS

Acarbose

Carbohydrates are broken down in the gut by a certain group of enzymes called *glucosidases*. One of these enzymes is called *alpha-glucosidase*. Acarbose stops this enzyme from working properly. Acarbose therefore delays carbohydrate absorption from the gut and reduces the rise in blood glucose levels following meals. Side effects include a bloating feeling, diarrhoea and flatulence. A newer agent, miglitol, is shorter acting and so may cause less side effects. It can be taken alone, or in combination with the other diabetes drugs.

Thiazolidinediones

Thiazolidinediones are sometimes called insulin sensitisers because they improve the action of insulin. They have no significant effect in the absence of insulin. Early studies have confirmed a lowering of blood glucose levels, no hypoglycemia and no weight gain. Clinical trials are in progress in Europe and the United States.

Conclusion

A recent estimate suggested that there are approximately half a million people with NIDDM in Australia. Most tend to be overweight at diagnosis and will initially be able to control their blood glucose levels with a diet/exercise program. In time, there is usually a progressive reduction in the amount of insulin produced by the pancreas and tablets are needed to control the blood glucose levels.

With further reductions in insulin secretion and consequent rises in blood glucose levels, insulin treatment may become necessary. Modern insulin treatment is simple, relatively cheap and effective. Weight gain is a problem, but this difficulty is far outweighed by the improved control of diabetes and the greater feeling of wellbeing.

Chapter 11

Hypoglycaemia

Hypoglycaemia is a word which means low blood glucose level and is commonly shortened to 'hypo'. It may occur in relation to the tablets and/or insulin used in treating diabetes. This chapter looks at what hypoglycaemia means: the symptoms, causes, and how to treat the problem if it occurs.

WHAT DOES HYPOGLYCAEMIA MEAN?

A 'hypo' occurs when the blood glucose level drops below the normal range. The normal range of blood glucose level is between 3.5 and 7 mmol/L. If the blood glucose level is low enough, it can cause specific symptoms. The level at which these symptoms occur can differ from person to person and at different times. Symptoms usually do not occur until the blood glucose level is 3 mmol/L or below, but this can vary. Hypoglycaemia occurs only in people treated with insulin and/or tablets, but not if diabetes is being treated with diet alone.

WHAT DOES IT FEEL LIKE TO HAVE HYPOGLYCAEMIA?

The symptoms that a person experiences during hypoglycaemia can appear quite quickly, or over several minutes. As the blood glucose level falls to approximately 3 mmol/L or lower, the early warning symptoms are experienced. There are really two types of symptoms. Some occur from there not being enough glucose for the brain to function properly; these include confusion, irritability, visual disturbance and headache. As the brain is able to recognise that the blood glucose is low, it sends out a message to the adrenal glands, which produce a substance called adrenaline. Adrenaline is a stress hormone and causes many of the symptoms characterising the beginning of a hypoglycaemic episode. Some adrenaline-related symptoms are sweating, shaking and trembling.

Symptoms of a hypoglycaemic episode

Adrenaline response

- feeling cold and sweaty
- shakiness/trembling
- feeling weak
- looking pale, with dilated pupils
- hunger
- palpitations

Not enough glucose to the brain

- inability to concentrate
- confusion
- headache
- visual disturbance
- irritability
- dizziness
- staggering, poor coordination
- tingling around the lips and mouth

Most people are able to recognise their own hypo symptoms easily, which can be different for each person. These symptoms can become very severe if ignored, or if neglected because the person is unaware of what they mean. For example, it can cause clumsiness and aggressive behaviour. If left to progress even further, it can lead to a convulsion (fit) or unconsciousness (coma), which may require medical help.

WHY DOES HYPOGLYCAEMIA HAPPEN?

All people with diabetes who are either taking insulin and/or taking tablets called sulphonylureas are at risk of having an episode of hypoglycaemia. Some of the most common reasons for a low blood glucose level are:

- not enough carbohydrate in the meals or missing a meal or a late meal;
- too much insulin or sulphonylurea tablets. this may be accidental;
- hypoglycaemia is more common when people have well-controlled blood glucose levels and so care may be necessary in such circumstances to achieve a satisfactory balance between the risk of hypoglycaemia and the degree of blood glucose control;

- drinking alcohol without food;
- more rapid absorption of insulin because the blood vessels dilate with heat or exercise and insulin is absorbed quickly, such as during hot weather, while exercising or while doing extra activities without eating extra carbohydrate foods or taking less insulin.

Reduced food intake can occur for many reasons. It may be due to being too busy at work to stop to eat, or the person may be having trouble keeping food down because of anxiety about an exam or job interview, or have an illness such as the flu and just not feel like eating very much.

Too much medication can be given accidentally by injecting too much insulin or, as sometimes can occur, having a double dose of tablets. This can happen when people forget that they took their medication earlier. Sometimes it can occur because of lifestyle change, e.g. going on that well-deserved holiday and relaxing. People can require less insulin than needed while working because relaxation is less stressful, although it may also be due to an increase in activity levels.

Undertaking extra activities or more exercise than normal burns up blood glucose. Exercise makes the insulin work better. Therefore, more glucose is taken up into the muscles in the body. This effect can continue for up to 15 hours after strenuous exercise or activity has occurred. Bruce Wainwright, in his book *Diabetic Rewards,* recalls a particular game of golf where:

> Without me suspecting that I was heading off the planet, I collapsed into a heap. At my turn, I took a swing and missed the ball and then another and then without a murmur fell to the ground. Golf has become a wonderful challenge. The exercise is great and what's more, there are no longer any low blood sugar problems. It certainly took a few games to make me realise how to cope.

As stated before, hypoglycaemia can occur for a lot of different reasons. It cannot always be avoided, but experience in planning and prevention, and the ability to recognise the symptoms early, enable the person to manage hypoglycaemic episodes appropriately.

HOW TO TREAT HYPOGLYCAEMIA WHEN IT OCCURS

The early warning symptoms of hypoglycaemia have been discussed. Now its treatment will be discussed. When a person recognises that he or she is experiencing hypoglycaemia, he or she should eat *one* of the choices given below:

7 jelly beans
3 glucose tablets (obtainable from the chemist)
$1/3$ of a can of soft drink (not diet or lo-cal)
2 heaped teaspoons of sugar or honey

A more substantial carbohydrate-containing food should then be eaten, e.g. 2 biscuits, or 1 slice of bread. If it is near to the time of the next meal or snack, then simply eat that meal or snack.

Never delay treating a hypoglycaemic episode; it must be treated straight away. By doing this, the blood glucose level will rise and the feelings or symptoms will go away over a short period of time, within 10–15 minutes.

It is essential for people with diabetes to carry food items with them to treat a hypo. Some people suggest carrying hypo treatments that they do not particularly like. The reasoning behind this is that, if the food is too tempting, when the hypo occurs, the food may no longer be there. It will have been eaten by the person with diabetes, or their children who have found the attractive food item. For this reason, it may be better to carry sugar sachets or glucose tablets.

Sometimes the symptoms (sweating, trembling etc.) of hypoglycaemia can be minimal or missed all together. This is known as hypoglycaemia unawareness. If this does happen, the effects of a low blood glucose level can become more serious so that the person suddenly becomes aggressive and/or their behaviour becomes inappropriate. If a friend, relative or partner does not help at this time, the episode can progress to unconsciousness or an epileptic fit. It is important that members of the family or close friends are aware of how to treat a hypo. They can be very helpful in recognising the early signs of hypoglycaemia and can tactfully help in early treatment.

The problem of hypoglycaemia unawareness tends to increase the longer a person has had insulin dependent diabetes (IDDM), but it may also be related to the frequency of low blood glucose levels. Recent research has shown that a low blood glucose level of, say, 3 mmol/L that does not upset the person (and may not be recognised except by a finger-prick measurement) will reduce the warning symptoms of another low blood glucose for the next 24 hours. So someone who is striving for good glucose control and having one or two blood glucose levels of around 3–4 mmol/L each day may be in a constant state of hypoglycaemia unawareness. A slight reduction in some of their insulin doses or adjustment of carbohydrate intake, with frequent blood glucose testing, may avoid many of these low blood glucose levels and restore symptoms. Hence, the person may find they can again recognise their hypos by feelings of sweating, trembling, tingling etc.

Most people who have diabetes are well able to recognise their symptoms of a low blood glucose. They are able to treat it quickly and simply with nobody else in the room even being aware of it having happened. For example:

> Jeffrey was in a business meeting when he felt the early warnings of hypoglycaemia — a little sweating, tremor and an intense hunger. No one noticed, there was an intense discussion going on around the table. He added 2 heaped teaspoons of sugar to his coffee and ate several plain, sweet biscuits from the tea tray in the midlle of the table. He was able to continue contributing to the meeting without anyone noticing his problem, by using readily available items to treat his hypo symptoms straight away.

Many people who have diabetes have a fear of hypoglycaemia. This fear can be because of an unpleasant experience in the past, or because of a story about what happened to someone else with diabetes who had a hypo. One woman I met had become terrified of having a hypoglycaemic episode, not because she had already experienced a bad hypo, but because she had never actually had one. Like many people, she had become fearful of hypoglycaemia simply because she did not know what to expect. Yet, other people may have a hypo once a week and experience no fear at all. They state that if they have a hypoglycaemic episode or feel early symptoms, they simply treat it. Unfortunately, no one can ever guarantee those who are fearful that they will never have a hypoglycaemic episode.

Quite often, people who have diabetes are made aware that they are having a hypo by a family member, partner or friend. Many people recognise the fact that their partner is able to pick up the signs before they can. It may be that their eyes have become glazed (dilated pupils), they are pale or sweaty, or that they have suddenly become argumentative. Of course, some family members may say that you are always argumentative! However, this characteristic usually becomes far more exaggerated than normal if someone is having a hypo. Many people are told by their partner that they need to eat something or to test their blood glucose level. On testing, they find the blood glucose level is 3 mmol/L, or less.

This demonstrates that it is very important that members of your family, your partner and your friends know about diabetes and what to do so they can help during a hypo. It is also important that they are given information about how to treat a hypoglycaemic episode. In that way, they will be able to help identify a hypo and, if needed, to provide the correct treatment.

Deciding to inform members of the family, workmates and friends is not always easy. People feel that friends and family can become overly concerned, i.e. watching them all the time for signs and watching what they eat or do. All this can make people feel so restricted in making decisions that they decide not to tell anyone at their new job, or not to tell new friends. For example:

> Sally decided not to tell any of her new workmates that she had diabetes. After working with them for several months, she had a severe hypo which caused her to become unconscious. No one was aware that she had diabetes and they were very upset when it happened. When the ambulance arrived, they found that she had a very low blood glucose level. If they had known, her workmates could have helped her by being aware of what to do. Sally explained everything subsequently and found people were helpful and supportive. Two of her workmates had someone in the family with diabetes!

Some people who have diabetes will choose not to tell everyone that they meet, but it is a good idea to let people who are close to you know. They can then learn what to do if help is needed in any particular situation.

WHAT IS GLUCAGON?

Glucagon is a hormone which is made naturally in the pancreas. It causes blood glucose levels to rise by releasing stores of glucose from the liver. Insulin, which is also made naturally in the pancreas, lowers blood glucose, as it helps the muscles of the body to use glucose as energy for everyday activities. These two hormones keep the blood glucose level very stable in people who do not have diabetes.

Glucagon can be used in people who have diabetes and are having a severe hypoglycaemic episode, i.e. are unable to swallow sweet drinks or are unconscious. When glucagon is injected, the liver releases its stored glucose into the bloodstream and the blood glucose level rises, enabling the individual to regain consciousness. The treatment of the hypoglycaemia can then be continued with carbohydrate foods as previously discussed.

Glucagon is available in injection form, like insulin. Glucagon is a safe drug as it is produced naturally by the body. Thus, an overdose of glucagon cannot occur and there are no major side effects from using it.

Glucagon is available from chemists. However, it is necessary to have a prescription from a doctor. The best way to learn how to use glucagon is by talking to a diabetes educator. The educator can show people with diabetes and/or a friend how to use glucagon, and discuss when its use is necessary.

Glucagon is injected into the body in the same way as insulin. It can be injected under the skin like insulin (subcutaneously) or into the muscle (intramuscularly) in the abdomen, arms, legs or buttocks. In fact, glucagon will work well if it is injected in just about any part of the body.

The person should wake up within 10–15 minutes. He or she must then have something to eat, again following the steps mentioned on page 84. If the person does not wake up, ring for an ambulance.

WHAT ARE THE BEST WAYS TO HELP PREVENT HYPOGLYCAEMIA?

Here are some precautions that may help in treating or preventing a hypoglycaemic eipsode.
- Carry some jelly beans or two sachets of sugar at all times if taking insulin or a sulphonylurea tablet, and eat these at the first symptoms of a hypo.
- Eat carbohydrate at every meal.
- Be careful to take the correct dose of insulin or tablets.

- Eat extra carbohydrate food before exercising and check blood glucose level afterwards. A low blood glucose level may occur for up to 15 hours after unusual vigorous exercise.
- Do not drink alcohol without eating.
- Know the profile of action of your tablets and/or insulin.
- Carry some identification that indicates that you have diabetes and the current treatment you are taking.
- Explain to colleagues, friends and relatives how to treat and recognise a hypoglycaemic episode, in case drowsiness or unconsciousness prevents you from treating the hypo yourself.
- Record hypoglycaemic episodes in a diary or journal. Discuss this record with a doctor and/or diabetes educator, as hypos can usually be prevented and should not occur on a regular basis. Treatment may need to be adjusted.
- When unable to eat usual meals, follow sick day routine (*see* chapter 12, 'The highs of diabetes').

WHAT IF UNCONSCIOUSNESS OCCURS?

- *Do not give food or drink to an unconscious person.*
- Roll the person onto their side.
- If it is available, inject 1 mg glucagon subcutaneously (under the skin) or into muscle tissue of the stomach, leg or arm. The glucagon should start having an effect within 15 minutes.
- Call the doctor or ambulance. They can give a concentrated glucose solution intravenously (into a vein).

Chapter 12

The Highs of Diabetes

HYPERGLYCAEMIA

What is hyperglycaemia? Hyperglycaemia means a high blood glucose level and usually refers to a glucose level above 15 mmol/L. Untreated high blood glucose levels can lead, in the short term, to feeling generally unwell and to infections, such as bladder infections or thrush (*Candida albicans*).

In the long term, if hyperglycaemia continues over a period of years, it can contribute to damage in several parts of the body, such as the eyes, kidneys, heart, circulation and nerves (*see* chapter 13, 'Avoiding long-term complications').

WHAT ARE THE MOST COMMON CAUSES OF HYPERGLYCAEMIA?

There are many reasons for developing high blood glucose levels. High blood glucose readings can occur when a person does not take enough diabetes medication, whether it is tablets or insulin. If the body's need for insulin increases at any time, high blood glucose levels are likely to result.

Stress is one reason for this increase, e.g. anxiety about family or work problems. Medical causes of hyperglycaemia include common illnesses, chest infection and some medications such as corticosteroids (prednisone, dexamethazone or cortisone — used for arthritis and asthma). This problem also arises when people eat more or decrease activity levels. For example:

Soon after Simone got a new job, she attended the diabetes service to get help with recent high blood glucose levels. The reason for her higher blood glucose readings was thought to be a combination of an increased amount of food containing fat and sugar, and stopping her regular gym class. She stopped getting a lot of food from the tea trolley at work and started back at the gym.

Excess alcohol may also have a deleterious affect on blood glucose levels (*see* chapter 21, 'Eating away from home' for safe use of alcohol).

WHAT DOES IT FEEL LIKE TO HAVE HYPERGLYCAEMIA?

As the blood glucose level rises, the following symptoms will occur:
- **Passing lots of urine**
  With high blood glucose levels, glucose spills over into the urine and drags additional water with it, increasing the amount of urine.
- **Dry mouth**
- **Excessive thirst**
  The increased amount of urine causes a lack of water in the body, which is sensed by the brain (in the hypothalamus), which in turn sends out a message to drink.
- **Blurred vision**
  High blood glucose levels increase the amount of glucose in the lens of the eye, which makes the lens swell and become less able to focus light in the retina.
- **Tiredness**
  Tiredness is due to such things as a lack of effective energy (because of a lack of insulin), a breakdown of protein in the muscle, dehydration and some body salt loss.

Some people do not feel all or even any of these symptoms of hyperglycaemia, perhaps because the blood glucose levels are not yet very high. However, if the high blood glucose is not treated in someone with insulin dependent diabetes meillitus (IDDM), vomiting, nausea and abdominal pain may develop. If still not treated appropriately, the person with IDDM can develop ketoacidosis (please read on for details). In those people who have non-insulin dependent diabetes (NIDDM), hyperosmolar coma is a possible risk.

IF I GET THIS PROBLEM, WHAT SHOULD I DO?

Look for the possible cause of the high glucose level – e.g. was the medication forgotten, is there an infection developing? People with IDDM should check urine for ketones. If ketones are present or an infection is brewing, contact should be made with the local doctor or diabetes service.

Check the blood glucose level (BGL) every 2–4 hours to see if it is improving. Drink enough fluid to satisfy thirst. If the BGL does not improve or vomiting occurs, sick day management (see pp 93–94) should be commenced and a doctor or diabetes service contacted. It may be unwise to exercise if the BGL is more than 15 mmol/L, as at this level the blood glucose may rise further.

KETONES AND KETOACIDOSIS

What are ketones?

- When there is not enough insulin in the body, the body breaks down fat for energy. As glucose is not entering the body's cells when there is a lack of insulin, glucose accumulates in the bloodstream.
- When fat is used as the energy source by cells, there are acidic by-products called ketones. Increasing levels of ketones can build up in the blood and some pass into the urine (these can be detected using a urine testing strip). Some ketone production can also occur with starvation, but this is only a small amount and quickly disappears upon eating and does not lead to severe illness.
- If there is a severe lack of insulin, which usually only occurs in IDDM, ketoacidosis can occur when blood glucose levels rise and ketones build up in the blood at the same time. Acidosis from ketones causes vomiting, which worsens the dehydration from the high blood glucose.
- Ketoacidosis can come on over 12 hours or more and is a serious medical problem which must be treated urgently.

Without treatment, the dehydration and acidosis will worsen and lead to coma.

What causes ketoacidosis and what does it feel like?

Ketoacidosis occurs when there is a major mismatch between the amount of insulin taken, e.g. a missed or inadequate dose given, and the amount of insulin needed by the body. The need for insulin is increased by illness or infection. It is a common mistake not to take insulin, or enough insulin, when someone is too sick to eat.

People with ketoacidosis usually have the symptoms of hyperglycaemia, as previously discussed, plus the following specific symptoms:

- a sweet sickly smell on the breath, like nail polish remover (acetone);
- nausea;
- abdominal pain; and
- vomiting.

A later, more severe stage causes deep sighing breathing, drowsiness and then coma.

How can ketoacidosis be prevented?

- Even when sick, it is essential for people with IDDM to take at least the usual dose of insulin. The body needs insulin to function properly even if the usual amounts of food cannot be eaten. It is possible that extra insulin may be required because the body's need for insulin can increase with illness.
- Even if nauseated, fluid intake is vital. Try taking small sips frequently. This helps to prevent dehydration.
- Carbohydrate should be taken even when not eating normally. Some people find it easier to drink flat non-diabetic lemonade (not the low-joule variety) when food cannot be kept down. See below.
- When you are ill, blood glucose levels should be measured every second hour until they have improved, and urine checked for ketones.
- It is essential to contact the doctor or diabetes educator if vomiting persists, fluids cannot be tolerated or the urine shows ketones.

DEALING WITH SICK DAYS

During illness, stress hormones such as adrenaline and cortisone are released in the body and make insulin less effective. This can causes blood glucose levels to rise. When a person has good diabetes control, the blood glucose level is usually between 4 and 8 mmol/L, with occasional increases up to 10 mmol/L (the acceptable range of fluctuation is greater in IDDM but it is desirable that most readings be between 4 and 10 mmol/L). When a person with diabetes becomes sick, even with a common ailment such as a cold or flu, the blood glucose level can increase markedly. It is therefore important to continue to take at least the usual dose of insulin during periods of illness. In fact, sometimes an increase in insulin may be necessary during illness. It is important to monitor the blood glucose levels as high blood glucose levels can interfere with the body's ability to fight infection and recover from illness. For example:

> Ronald contacted the diabetes service. He sounded unwell on the phone. Ronald explained that he had the flu, had vomited once and had mild diarrhoea. He was worried how this would affect his diabetes.
>
> Following advice, Ronald tested his blood glucose levels and his urine for ketones. His blood glucose was 15 mmol/L, but he had no ketones in his urine. Ronald was able to manage his own care at home because he was able to keep fluids down and keep in regular telephone contact with the diabetes service. He was following the advice provided. This advice is outlined below.

Steps to follow when ill

- Check the blood glucose levels every 2 hours.
- People with IDDM should test urine for ketones every 6 hours.
- When ill, the person with diabetes should continue to take the diabetes tablets and/or insulin. Increased medication may be ordered by the doctor to control blood glucose levels and avoid ketones developing. Sometimes it is necessary to take extra small injections of quick-acting insulin every 2–3 hours until a very high blood glucose level is brought down to more reasonable levels.

- Be kind to your body. Drink plenty of fluids and ensure adequate rest.
- If the appetite is poor and regular meals cannot be eaten, replace meals with soft foods or nourishing drinks. The following foods may be tried:
  - puréed fruit ($2/3$ cup);
  - ice cream (4 tablespoons);
  - low-fat yoghurt (200 g);
  - unsweetened custard ($1/2$ cup) and banana ($1/2$);
  - soup, plus toast or bread ($1/2$ slice)
  - mashed potato, rice or porridge ($1/2$ cup); and
  - biscuits (2) or toast/bread (1 slice).
- Avoid spicy and fatty foods.
- If there is vomiting and/or diarrhoea, fluids containing sugar or honey will provide the body with the energy it needs and will also help prevent hypoglycaemia. Avoid milk-based products as they can worsen diarrhoea. A half to one cup each hour of the following fluids may be tried: fruit juice; 'flat' non-diabetic soft drinks, e.g. lemonade; non-diabetic cordial; non-diabetic jelly; tea plus 2 heaped teaspoons of sugar; or lemon juice with water plus 2 teaspoons of honey.

When to see the doctor

- Contact the doctor if any of the following are present:
- Vomiting and/or diarrhoea persists.
- The blood glucose levels rise above 15 mmol/L.
- Ketones are present in the urine.
- No fluids can be tolerated.
- There is severe thirst or drowsiness.
- The illness does not improve.
- There is uncertainty about what to do.

MEDICAL INVESTIGATIONS OR OPERATIONS

When people with diabetes need special medical tests requiring a period of abstinence from food (fasting), it is advisable to the contact the doctor or educator about how to manage the diabetes. Always inform the pathologist or x-ray specialist doing the test when making the initial arrangements that you have diabetes. It is preferable to have the earliest appointment in the day for the test to be done. The blood glucose level is usually checked before the procedure and medication may need to be adjusted, under the guidance of the doctor or diabetes service.

When admitted to hospital for an operation, the person with NIDDM may require insulin therapy temporarily because the body's insulin requirement usually increases during this time. Also, on admission, let the ward staff know that you have diabetes so that appropriate meals and monitoring can be arranged. For people already receiving insulin therapy prior to admission to hospital, the insulin regimen may need to be altered for a short period. During surgery, it is vital to avoid hypoglycaemia, as it is difficult to detect during anaesthesia and could be missed. At the time of surgery and in the period after the operation, it is usually the aim of the doctors to keep the blood glucose levels between and 5 and 12 mmol/L. In keeping them in this range, diabetes control is optimised and the body's tissues have the best opportunity to heal without infection.

Chapter 13

Avoiding Long-term Complications

In this chapter, the potential long-term complications of diabetes mellitus are described. Simple guidelines for avoiding these complications are also provided.

CHECKLIST TO PREVENT DIABETIC COMPLICATIONS

1. Achieve and maintain good blood glucose control.
2. Have regular reviews with an eye specialist.
3. Have your blood pressure checked regularly.
4. Do not smoke.
5. Practise simple daily foot care, including inspecting and moisturising the feet.
6. Attend a podiatrist regularly if there is nerve or circulation damage in the feet, or if you are elderly.
7. Exercise regularly and keep your weight as near ideal as possible.

Most people with diabetes first hear about the possibility of developing complications not long after the diagnosis is made. Unfortunately, as this is usually a time of some stress, the correct medical information may be confused with the more dramatic stories told by friends and relatives. However, to carry out long-term changes in lifestyle in order to prevent the development of diabetic complications, it is essential to know first what damage can occur as a result of poorly controlled diabetes and then how it can be avoided.

This chapter describes the possible long-term damage and then gives a simple preventative regimen suitable for daily life.

HIGH BLOOD GLUCOSE LEVELS ARE THE MAJOR CULPRIT

Even now, the exact processes by which high blood glucose damages body tissues are not fully understood. The damage takes years to develop and several factors can play a part. However, there is now proof that in the majority of problems caused by diabetes, high blood glucose is a major cause. To avoid such damage, it is necessary to the maintain blood glucose level as close as possible to normal (*see* chapter 3, 'Achieving good diabetes control: why and how').

THE AREAS OF THE BODY WHICH CAN BE DAMAGED

The major sites of potential damage are the eyes, the kidneys, the nerves and the large arteries. This chapter deals with each area separately.

Diabetic retinopathy: the causes

When long-term blood glucose control is poor, small blood vessels carrying oxygen and food to the back of the eye (retina) become blocked. While fragile new blood vessels form to replace them, the new vessels are very prone to breakage and bleeding. While these events are happening, there are no symptoms and the vision remains normal. The only way to find out if these early changes are occurring is to have a full examination of the back of the eye, using drops to dilate the pupil and an ophthalmoscope (an instrument to shine light at the back of the eye).

This eye check-up should be done by an ophthalmologist, usually at least every 2 years. If abnormalities are seen, it is sometimes useful to inject dye into a vein in the arm and have a photograph made of the retinal blood vessels as the dye goes through them (fluorescein angiogram). This shows areas of blood vessel blockages or leakage of dye from abnormal vessels.

If not treated, and blood glucose levels remain high, the blood vessel damage will continue. Uncontrolled high blood pressure can also worsen the damage. The resulting bleeding can lead to permanent scarring of the retina. Sudden symptoms of loss of vision often come late in the process, when some irreversible damage has already occurred.

Diabetic retinopathy: prevention and treatment

1. Excellent control of blood glucose levels prevents diabetic retinopathy (*see* Chapter 3, 'Achieving good diabetes control: why and how').
2. Regular eye review, preferably by an ophthalmologist (eye specialist), is essential. As there are no symptoms, the only means of diagnosing the early changes of diabetic damage is by full examination of the eyes, preferably by an eye specialist. Young people with IDDM should start this 6 years after diagnosis. Although the damage takes years to develop, people with non-insulin dependent diabetes mellitus (NIDDM) may have had diabetes for years without knowing it, and therefore should begin eye review at diagnosis.
3. Laser therapy can be used to treat already damaged areas. Laser therapy consists of a very intense light beam being focused on the damaged areas at the back of the eye to 'burn' them away, thus preventing secondary growth of weak, new vessels. This procedure is done as an outpatient, often over several sessions, without the need for hospitalisation or a general anaesthetic. There can be some discomfort and the vision is often blurred for a couple of hours afterwards, but the benefits are great.

Cataracts: the cause

The clear lens of the eye works just like that in a camera, focusing incoming light onto the retina. If the lens becomes cloudy or milky, it cannot let light through properly and this gradually makes the vision blurry. This clouding of the lens is called a cataract. Cataracts develop with increasing age in many people, but high blood glucose levels increase the likelihood. This occurs because there is an accumulation, or trapping, of a by-product of glucose called *sorbitol* in the lens when the blood glucose is high. In the short term, the trapped sorbitol attracts water into the lens and causes swelling of the lens, producing the blurring of vision which often accompanies high blood glucose levels. However, this is reversible after a few weeks of good blood glucose control. In the long term, repeated swelling damages the lens permanently, causing cataracts.

Cataracts: Prevention and treatment

1. Excellent control of blood glucose levels lessens the chance of cataract formation.
2. When the cataract is causing loss of vision, the usual treatment is to remove the whole lens and replace it immediately with a plastic one. This procedure can be done as a day-only patient, often using a local anaesthetic. A long-wear contact lens or thick glass lenses can be used instead of the implant if there is a problem with the implant.

The kidneys: diabetic nephropathy

Persistently high blood glucose levels can damage the small blood vessels in the kidney. The kidneys are filters and their ability to filter the blood adequately can be lessened with long-term poor control. Before permanent damage has occurred, minute amounts of a protein, albumin, can be found in the urine using a special test (microalbumin test). Usually, the person experiences no symptoms and is unaware of kidney disease until substantial damage has occurred. High blood pressure often accompanies and worsens the kidney disease.

If poor blood glucose control continues, permanent kidney damage can result, with leakage of large amounts of protein in the urine. If damage continues for years, some people will experience kidney failure. People can then develop fluid retention from loss of albumin from the blood. Eventually, there may be a need for dialysis three times a week to clean the blood (or, alternatively, regular flushing of fluid via a catheter into the abdominal cavity – peritoneal dialysis). Some people may then be able to have a kidney transplant, but must take cortisone-like drugs for life to suppress rejection. People with IDDM already having a kidney transplant may be considered for a pancreatic transplant at the same time (*see* chapter 24, 'Research in diabetes mellitus').

Prevention and treatment

1. Achieve and maintain excellent blood glucose control.
2. Have blood pressure measured regularly and treated if necessary.
3. Have urine tested for microalbumin annually.

High blood pressure (hypertension)

While high blood pressure is quite common throughout the general community, diabetes increases the chances of developing it even further. Many years of pumping the blood through the body at high pressures can damage the heart and the blood vessels, eventually causing heart failure, heart attacks or strokes.

Prevention and treatment

1. Have blood pressure measured regularly.
2. If blood pressure is persistently high (greater than 160/90 at three check-ups), treatment should usually begin with the following lifestyle changes:
   – weight loss;
   – salt restriction;
   – exercise; and
   – stress reduction.

If blood pressure still requires treatment after a trial of lifestyle changes, the usual recommended type of drug for first-line treatment is what is called an ACE inhibitor. ACE inhibitors are drugs which have been shown to have a kidney protecting effect. However, as with all drugs, there are sometimes side effects, most commonly a dry cough. Other drugs can be used as well, particularly a group of drugs called calcium channel blockers. Drug treatment is usually needed for life, but losing weight may reduce or, in milder cases, eliminate the need for drug treatment. It is important to check that the tablet you take is appropriate for someone with diabetes.

Atherosclerosis

Atherosclerosis (thickening and then narrowing of the large arteries in the body) occurs in everyone as we age. This process can lead to heart disease, strokes and poor leg circulation. Having diabetes can increase the risk of atherosclerosis, particularly in premenopausal women, who are otherwise at relatively low risk.

The major factors which contribute to the arterial narrowing are smoking, high blood pressure, a high cholesterol level, high triglyceride levels, obesity, a family history of heart disease, diabetes and lack of exercise. Whether stress also plays a part remains controversial.

Heart disease

If arteries to the heart (coronary arteries) are becoming blocked, people often experience chest pain on exercise, which stops when the activity stops. This is called *angina*. It is usually a heavy, crushing pain. A heart attack occurs when there is a sudden, more complete blockage of a coronary artery. In this case, there is usually severe chest pain unrelated to exercise, often with sweating and paleness of the skin, and lasting for some hours.

Poor leg circulation

If the leg arteries are narrowed by arteriosclerosis, the usual symptom is severe calf pain on walking, which disappears on stopping. The poor circulation can also contribute to poor healing of infections or ulcers on the feet. The feet tend to be cold, pale and hairless.

Poor brain circulation

If the brain arteries are narrowed, temporary 'mini-strokes' can occur – i.e. temporary loss of movement in one arm or difficulty with speech. A more severe blockage gives a permanent stroke, e.g. causing permanent weakness or loss of feeling down one side, loss of speech or balance. The mini strokes are often a warning that a major stroke is imminent. All the arteries can be examined by special x-rays with dye injections to outline where the blockages are.

Atherosclerosis: prevention and treatment

1. Not smoking is a major positive factor in preventing atherosclerosis. It is of major health benefit for a person with diabetes mellitus to stop smoking: damage to the arteries will be much less likely, without even considering the prevention of damage to other organs.
2. Blood pressure should be checked regularly and, if persistently high (greater than 160/90), it should be treated.
3. Fasting cholesterol and triglyceride levels (blood fat levels) should be measured and dietary and lifestyle change begun if the tests are abnormal. Drug treatment may be necessary if lifestyle changes involving a low-fat diet, weight control and exercise do not lower the blood fats satisfactorily. Different

drugs are used depending on whether it is the cholesterol or triglyceride level which is most elevated.
4. Symptoms such as chest or calf pain on exercise or exertion should be reported to the doctor for assessment.
5. Regular exercise such as walking is beneficial, using appropriate footwear and making small increases in quantity over time. The benefits of exercise are multiple, and weight and blood fat levels can also improve (*see* chapter 7, 'Exercise').
6. Optimise body weight (*see* chapter 5, 'Introduction to food'). It is usually best to keep weight in the normal healthy range. Discuss this with your doctor and dietitian. For the overweight, drug therapy may be of benefit when taken as part of a combined approach to losing weight. Currently, dexfenfluramine is recommended for 3 months' use at a time. Other drugs will be available in the future.

If atherosclerosis is producing symptoms, various forms of treatment may be needed in addition.
1. DRUG THERAPY. Several drugs are used to prevent or treat atherosclerosic symptoms, one of which is a low-dose aspirin.
2. ANGIOPLASTY. In some cases, the narrowing of arteries can be widened from within by a balloon being threaded in and blown up to open out the narrowed area and then withdrawn.
3. BYPASS OPERATION. Severely narrowed arteries can be bypassed to get around the obstruction(s) using grafts of other blood vessels, such as leg veins. This operation is used to bypass blockages in the heart, legs and to the brain.

Foot complications: diabetic peripheral neuropathy

Long-term poor control of blood glucose levels can damage the nerves of the body, particularly those supplying feeling to the feet. Less commonly, the hands or other areas of the body are also affected.

Diabetic peripheral neuropathy

Neuropathy usually causes numbness and sometimes burning or pins and needles in the feet, particularly at night in bed. As numb feet are more liable to deformities which then result in areas of high foot pressure, calluses (hard skin) form at such pressure areas and can crack and become infected. Also, the skin is often dry and fissures can form at the heels. With numbness of the feet, there is also a risk that injuries may not be noticed (unless feet are inspected daily). Infection can then enter through unnoticed breaks in the skin and, if there is also poor circulation, healing can be slow. Foot ulcers can be the result of these problems and hospitalisation with intravenous antibiotic treatment is sometimes necessary to achieve adequate healing. There may be a need for surgery to remove dead tissue. Excessive alcohol intake doubles the likelihood of developing neuropathy.

Prevention and treatment

1. Excellent diabetes control helps prevent diabetic neuropathy.
2. Drink alcohol within safe levels.
3. A regular daily foot care routine is essential if neuropathy is present (*see* chapter 14,'Foot care').
4. If there is neuropathy or poor circulation to the legs, regular podiatry is necessary.

Regular podiatry is recommended for all people with diabetes, but is essential for those with peripheral neuropathy, poor leg circulation or a previous foot ulcer. Podiatrists deal with foot problems, trimming thick or misshapen nails and safely treating corns and calluses. They advise on footwear and can make orthotics for shoes to help correct foot deformities (*see* chapter 14, 'Foot care').

Autonomic neuropathy

Rarely, the nerves which affect the automatic body functions are also damaged by poor diabetes control. This is called *autonomic neuropathy*. If this affects the bowel, there can be slow absorption of food from the stomach, or disorganised bowel function, sometimes giving diarrhoea at night time. Bladder function can also be affected, with inadequate bladder emptying and subsequent urinary tract infection. If blood pressure regulation is affected, there can be dizziness due to a drop in blood pressure when standing up. These conditions all need to be investigated by a specialist, who can help with treatment designed to relieve symptoms.

Chapter 14

Foot Care

This chapter outlines how to preserve a pair of feet for a lifetime. Ask yourself, 'How far would I get without both my feet and how would I cope with life?' That may sound a little dramatic, but diabetic complications of the feet, e.g. ulcers, are responsible for more time spent in hospital than any other complication of diabetes. In severe cases, foot complications can lead to the loss of a limb. Many of the foot problems associated with diabetes are caused by poor circulation and a lack of sensation in the feet (*see* chapter 13, 'Avoiding long-term complications').

The good news is that many foot problems are easily preventable with a few minutes of your time spent checking your feet each day, an increased awareness of your feet and a good daily foot care routine. Unfortunately, feet are the most neglected parts of the body. If I had a dollar for every patient who came into my surgery and said that their feet were dry, and then admitted they apply moisturiser to the body but stop at the ankles, I would be a rich woman. How about we clean up our act and start to give our feet the tender, loving care they deserve? Remember, Prevention is better than cure. Let's look at the steps to take to prevent problems arising.

FOOT CARE ROUTINE

If you want to help to maintain your feet in a healthy state, it is essential that you develop a good daily foot care routine. The following tips are a guide:

1. Wash your feet in warm water using a mild, unperfumed soap. When getting into a bath, test the temperature of the water with your hand first as you may have numbness (neuropathy) in the feet and can scald them if the water is too hot. Do not soak your feet unless you have been instructed to do so.

Soaking can rob the skin of some of its moisture (oils) and can make the skin less resistant to infection.
2. Dry your feet well, paying particular attention to the skin in between your toes. Moisture left in between the toes can lead to tinea, infection and the skin splitting. If necessary, swab in between toes with methylated spirits to dry them properly.
3. Apply a moisturiser all over your feet to keep the skin supple, avoiding the area in between the toes.
4. Look at your feet thoroughly every day. Always remember that you may have a lack of sensation or numbness of the feet caused by diabetes and any foot problems may not be painful. Examining your feet daily is a very important aspect of preventing foot problems. Check in between the toes, under the soles of the feet and around the backs of the heels. If you are unable to get down to the feet, place a mirror on the floor (in a good light) and then place your feet at such an angle that you can view the soles of your feet. Ask a friend or relative to help you if your eyesight is poor. When examining your feet look for:
   – any splits in the skin;
   – discharge;
   – discoloration; and
   – signs of infection, e.g. warmth, redness or swelling.

It is important to remember that, when you have diabetes, you are more prone to developing an infection in your feet. Something as simple as neglecting to cut your toenails for an unreasonable length of time can have disastrous consequences for a person with diabetes. For example:

> Betty developed a problem on her toe due to the long toenail cutting into the flesh of the adjoining toe. This situation could easily have been prevented. It was only detected when the toes were separated and examined. With the nail cut and protection of the toe, healing was rapid.

CUTTING TOENAILS

If you suffer from ingrown toenails, fungal nails or thick, misshapen nails, you need to consult your podiatrist for nail trimming and advice.

When cutting your toe nails the following rules apply:
1. Cut your toenails straight across (no fancy shapes, please) and file any sharp edges.
2. Avoid cutting the nails too sharp and do not cut them down at the sides as this may cause them to ingrow.
3. Do not poke anything sharply down the sides of the nails, as you may break the skin and start an infection.
4. Always use clean nail clippers. Wipe them with methylated spirits before and after use and store them in a clean, dry place. Please do not be tempted to use the garden secateurs or the dog's nail clippers.

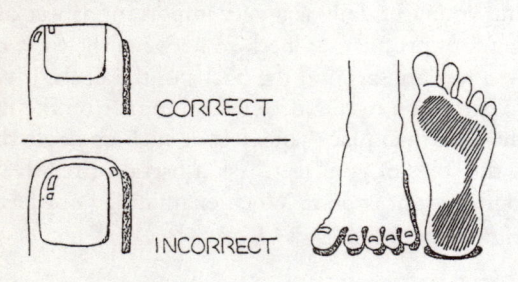

CORNS AND CALLUSES

When examining your feet, you may notice corns or hard, callused skin on the feet. Do not perform 'bathroom surgery' on these lesions. Over the years, I have seen many patients who have been referred to our podiatry clinic by the hospital accident and emergency department after performing corn and callus removals with razor blades, corn pads, corn paints etc.

Home cures can often lead to infection and ulceration of the feet and result in a much bigger problem than the initial corn or callus. Many of the proprietary corn and wart paints contain an acid which can burn the skin and cause severe problems such as ulcers on the feet. Please seek professional advice and treatment for corns and calluses.

TINEA

Tinea, 'athletes foot', 'foot rot', whatever name you choose to call it, is a fungal infection of the skin and nails. Tinea is more common in the summer months when the weather is hot and humid, and the feet become sweaty. The favourite site for a fungal infection is in between the toes — an area often overlooked when it comes to drying the feet after showering.

To prevent tinea, good daily hygiene is essential. It is important to change your shoes and socks daily. Whenever possible, choose natural fibres for footwear to allow your feet to breathe. Tinea manifests itself as itchy, peeling skin with small blister-like eruptions or may cause white, soggy skin with splits in between the toes. If you notice symptoms of tinea, use a tinea preparation on the affected area until the symptoms disappear. It is also important to treat footwear with an antifungal powder to prevent re-infection. If the symptoms persist, seek professional advice. Left untreated, tinea can lead to further problems such as cellulitis.

Sometimes, when fungal infections are well established and involve nails, it may be necessary to take tablets of a special antibiotic active against fungi.

FIRST AID

One of the most important steps you can take to maintain good foot health is to purchase a first aid or foot care kit (available from Diabetes Australia, NSW).

Remember that, with diabetes, you may have a lack of sensation in your feet caused by damage to the nerves and therefore an injury such as a cut may not be painful. Your feet may also be slow to heal and it is essential that you carry out first aid measures promptly to prevent serious problems arising.

1. Wash and dry the affected area.
2. Apply an antiseptic to the wound.
3. Use a nonstick sterile dressing to cover the area.
4. Fix the dressing with a non-allergenic tape.
5. Change the dressing daily.

If the wound does not heal, seek advice from your GP or podiatrist.

FOOTWEAR

Your feet work very hard during your lifetime and deserve well-fitting, comfortable shoes. A large percentage of the foot problems we see arise from people wearing ill-fitting and unsuitable footwear. Your feet can change shape and size as you get older, so it is important to check that you are wearing the correct-sized shoes.

1. Buy new shoes in the afternoon as your feet tend to swell during the day.
2. Select well-fitting shoes and make sure you compare your foot shape (long/narrow, short/broad) to the shoe shape.
3. When buying new shoes, always feel inside the shoe for seams, stitching or anything that may cause an irritation to your feet.
4. Select the widest and lowest heels possible for greater stability.
5. Always wear shoes appropriate to the occasion – do not go bushwalking in sandals.
6. Do not wear your new shoes home from the shop. Always break them in gently at home before wearing them for a lengthy period. Start with half an hour to an hour per day, and inspect your feet afterwards for signs of rubbing or pressure.

Remember, prevention is better than cure.
It is important to protect your feet at all times with good, well-fitting shoes.

THE ROLE OF THE PODIATRIST

Podiatry is concerned with the diagnosis, prevention and treatment of foot disorders. The podiatrist plays a vital role in helping to maintain your feet in a healthy state. Everyone with diabetes should have an initial appointment with a podiatrist for an assessment of the feet. The podiatrist will then ascertain whether an annual check-up is indicated or more regular treatments are necessary for a specific problem.

On your first visit, the podiatrist will observe you walking into the surgery. He or she will then take a complete medical history. The podiatrist will look at your footwear as well as your feet, to check for any unusual wear patterns which may indicate an abnormal foot function.

Any bony abnormalities and superficial lesions such corns and calluses on your feet are noted. The circulation is assessed by feeling the pulses in your feet and observing the skin texture, colour and temperature. This may be followed by an assessment of the sensation in your feet using such instruments as a tuning fork, a percussion hammer or a monofilament.

The podiatrist will then treat any problems such as thick nails or fungal infections, and painlessly remove any corns or calluses. The cause of problems such as corns needs to be identified and addressed.

If you have problems with the way your foot functions, e.g. flat feet, the podiatrist will assess the mechanical function of your foot and probably suggest the appropriate therapy such as arch supports, orthoses or alterations to your shoes.

HELPFUL HINTS FOR HEALTHY FEET

1. Do not walk barefoot — always protect your feet.
2. Avoid anything that will restrict the circulation to your feet, such as tight garters, girdles, tight stockings or tight socks.
3. Avoid extremes of temperature.
4. Do not smoke.
5. Exercise regularly.
6. Always test the bath water with your hand first.
7. Do not sit too close to heaters or fires.
8. Have a regular podiatry check-up.

Note: For further information, please contact the branch of the Australian Podiatry Association in your state.

Chapter 15

Fertility and Pregnancy

There have been many advances in diabetes and pregnancy management since diabetes in pregnancy was first recognised in 1882, when only 22 cases had been reported. In those early days, women with insulin dependent diabetes mellitus (IDDM) were discouraged from becoming pregnant. However, the treatment of diabetes in general and diabetes in pregnancy in particular was revolutionised in 1921 with the discovery of insulin. Today, with careful planning, a woman with diabetes can expect an excellent outcome for herself and her child.

Pregnancy is always a challenge for the mother-to-be, and this is particularly so for the woman with diabetes. The situation is quite different for women with IDDM compared with those women who are diagnosed with gestational diabetes. Gestational diabetes is a form of diabetes which occurs only during pregnancy and this will be discussed as a separate topic later in this chapter. First of all, we will look at pregnancy in women with IDDM.

FERTILITY

In the early days of insulin therapy, when many women with IDDM were poorly controlled, amenorrhoea (absent menstruation) and low fertility were commonplace. Fortunately, women with IDDM whose diabetes is well controlled should now have approximately normal fertility rates. There is some evidence that diabetic women are slightly less fertile, possibly due to the more common occurrence of an irregular menstrual cycle and an increased risk of pelvic inflammatory disease. Infertility itself is a relatively common problem in the whole community (affecting an estimated 10% of all couples) and it can occur for a variety of reasons. Any severe illness can affect fertility and, in the case of someone with long-term IDDM, severe kidney disease may reduce fertility. Very rarely, an early menopause occurs in women in association with diabetes via a similar mechanism to the one that caused the diabetes (i.e. auto-immune destruction of the ovaries).

Most importantly, since fertility is generally normal in women with IDDM, pre-pregnancy planning is a crucial part of the management of pregnancy. With excellent blood glucose control at the time of conception, a woman with diabetes can expect to have a normal pregnancy and a healthy baby.

IDDM AND PREGNANCY

What does pregnancy do to diabetes control?

Pregnancy tends to make the blood glucose rise due to the hormones of pregnancy opposing the action of insulin. This usually means that increased insulin doses are needed. The action of insulin is particularly affected in mid-pregnancy (second trimester), when the levels of some pregnancy-related hormones rise (such as progesterone, cortisol, prolactin and placental lactogen), making the body more insulin resistant.

Risk to the mother

Today, the misfortune of a mother dying as a result of a pregnancy is extremely unlikely (occuring in less than 2 per 10,000 pregnancies). This figure may be slightly higher in diabetic women due to rare events such as diabetic ketoacidosis or severe toxaemia (eclampsia), but it is still a very rare event.

Risk to the baby

After the discovery of insulin in the 1920s, it became clear that the ordinary standard of diabetes control in non-pregnant diabetic women with diabetes was not good enough once they were pregnant. There was still a higher than usual rate of perinatal (throughout the pregnancy) deaths and congenital malformations. Although the precise cause of the excess stillbirths in IDDM still remains unknown, if the mother's blood glucose levels are kept within the normal range, it very rarely occurs. Half of the perinatal deaths are due to stillbirths and are usually associated with poor blood glucose control throughout the pregnancy. If diabetic ketoacidosis occurs, the baby can die; a low blood glucose level (hypoglycaemia) in the mother, however, does not seem to have an effect on the baby.

The incidence of congenital malformations in diabetic pregnancy is still up to 7%, which is three times higher than in the general population. The defects associated with IDDM include heart and skeletal malformations. They are believed to be due to poor diabetic control in the time around conception and during formation of the foetal organs (the first couple of months of pregnancy). This lack of good control generally occurs before the pregnancy has even been discovered. The possible role of hypoglycaemia has been examined extensively and there is no evidence that it has an effect on the baby. Cigarette smoking, which is strongly discouraged in any pregnancy, may act with diabetes to further increase the risk of malformations in the foetus.

Women with diabetes tend to have bigger (both larger and heavier) babies. This is mainly due to the higher amounts of glucose in the blood available to the baby. Higher than normal blood glucose levels stimulate the baby's pancreatic cells so that they secrete extra insulin, which causes the baby to grow bigger in the uterus. Paradoxically, extremely high blood glucose levels (greater than 20 mmol/L) may stop foetal insulin secretion and the baby may then be smaller than usual. The major problem resulting from a big baby is difficult delivery and, in some cases, vaginal delivery may not be possible because of the large size of the baby.

Other problems that are a little more likely to occur in the newborn babies of women with diabetes include: respiratory distress syndrome, low blood glucose levels, low calcium levels and jaundice. Respiratory distress syndrome is a breathing disorder of prematurity and its increased incidence in diabetic women is believed to be due to the high blood glucose and insulin levels which appear to slow down lung maturation. Hypoglycaemia in the baby after delivery is usually mild and short-lived, and can occur in the big babies who have been needing to produce extra insulin in the womb to deal with a high blood glucose from the mother. This is due to the continuing secretion of insulin from the baby's pancreas, which may have been further stimulated if high blood glucose levels occurred about the time of labour.

PREGNANCY MANAGEMENT IN IDDM

Careful planning and a close link with a medical team are important for the best outcome for both mother and child. Tight control of diabetes must begin before conception. This significantly reduces any risk of a major congenital defect. Good control needs to be maintained throughout the pregnancy to avoid the problems associated with having a big baby.

PRE-PREGNANCY

It is best to achieve excellent control of blood glucose levels for at least 3 months prior to conception. Women should aim to have a normal HbA1c, fasting or before-meal blood glucose level in the range of 3–6 mmol/L and levels less than 8 mmol/L following meals. This degree of control has been associated with a significant reduction in congenital malformations. On the other hand, with such tight control, there is usually an increased risk of hypoglycaemia. Although hypoglycaemia does not affect the foetus, it can clearly be dangerous to the expectant mother, e.g. while driving, swimming or cooking at the stove with young children about. Frequent monitoring of blood glucose levels and a good understanding of hypoglycaemia management are essential to minimise the risks of hypoglycaemia (*see* chapter 4, 'Assessment of diabetes control').

To achieve this degree of control, home blood glucose monitoring is essential (three to four tests/day) and usually three to four injections of insulin a day are needed. During this time, regular insulin dose adjustments are often required with the help of an endocrinologist or diabetes nurse educator. Insulin pumps are used rarely in Australia because they are expensive and are associated with some side effects. Pumps are only used in situations where it has been very difficult to achieve satisfactory control with other means.

It is a good idea to have a dietary review before the pregnancy. The aims are to achieve ideal body weight before pregnancy, to be aware of the nutrition requirements in pregnancy and to help in gaining good blood glucose control. Folic acid supplementation is generally recommended to all pregnant women to reduce the risk of neural tube defects.

Prior to conception, an eye specialist review is strongly recommended. If it is needed, fluorescein angiography should be performed before pregnancy as it is contra-indicated during pregnancy because of the dye injection which is used. Mild or background retinopathy is not a contra-indication to pregnancy as it can improve with good glucose control during pregnancy; however, if there is more severe or proliferative retinopathy, it must be treated before pregnancy occurs. A review of kidney function and blood pressure is also advised before conception, particularly in women who have eye disease because of the increased likelihood of accompanying kidney disease. Consultation with an obstetrician is also recommended at this stage. If there is a question of heart disease being present, an electrocardiograph (ECG) should be performed before conception, together with evaluation by a cardiologist.

ANTE-NATAL PERIOD

Once pregnancy is confirmed, women need to continue with frequent blood glucose monitoring. Often the insulin dose needs to be changed; sometimes a reduction in insulin dose is necessary early on in the pregnancy. However, more often than not, the dose needs to be slowly increased as the pregnancy progresses (due to an increase in the placental hormones which may make the body more insulin resistant). Regular review by the health care team is advised (weekly to fortnightly in the last couple of months).

Since tight blood glucose control is essential, there is an increased risk of hypoglycaemia at this time. It is therefore important that women with diabetes eat regularly and always carry quick-acting carbohydrate (*see* chapter 9). Glucagon should be readily available and family members should be trained in how to give it if necessary (*see* chapter 9).

Regular obstetric review is also necessary to monitor blood pressure, as well as the baby's growth and maturity. An eye review is recommended, particularly in women with any pre-existing eye disease. After 32 weeks' gestation, a weekly review is necessary to check blood pressure and the baby's growth. An ultrasound examination is usually performed at least once to assess the baby's size.

THE DELIVERY

Previously, the babies of women with diabetes were delivered quite early. Now, however, with improved diabetes control, pregnancy can proceed closer to full term, although early delivery can still be recommended for other medical reasons. Caesarean section is only performed if there are obstetric complications, not simply because of the presence of diabetes.

During delivery, blood glucose levels are monitored closely to prevent the mother from having high blood glucose levels, which predispose the baby to hypoglycaemia after delivery. With a planned induction of delivery, blood glucose levels are usually easily managed with low doses of insulin and an intravenous dextrose infusion. As soon as the baby is delivered, insulin can be ceased as the insulin needs fall dramatically in the first 24 hours after delivery. Following this period, something near to the usual insulin treatment before pregnancy is recommended.

POST-DELIVERY

The baby should be examined by a paediatrician and monitored for low blood glucose levels for 1–2 days. Hypoglycaemia occurs in 15–20% of babies born to mothers with diabetes. It usually responds to early feeding, but sometimes an intravenous glucose infusion may be necessary. There are usually no problems with breastfeeding provided the mother's carbohydrate intake is increased sufficiently to cover the carbohydrate being lost in the milk.

GESTATIONAL DIABETES MELLITUS

Gestational diabetes mellitus means diabetes developed during pregnancy and it is usually a temporary form of diabetes which is most often diagnosed between weeks 24 and 28 of the pregnancy. Approximately 3% of all pregnant women are affected by it in Australia. It develops in response to the increased levels of some hormones during pregnancy which oppose the action of insulin. Women who are at increased risk of developing diabetes later in life have a high risk of having gestational diabetes. Risk factors include: family history of diabetes, obesity, history of large babies (greater than 4 kg) and being more than 30 years old. However, gestational diabetes often occurs in women without any of these risk factors, so many experts now recommend that testing for diabetes is carried out in all pregnant women. If gestational diabetes mellitus has occurred in a previous pregnancy, it is likely to recur, but it is not inevitable.

SCREENING AND DIAGNOSIS

It is advised that pregnant women be tested for gestational diabetes between weeks 24 and 28 of the pregnancy, when diabetes is most likely to be apparent. Detecting it at this time also allows time for treatment. Women at higher risk of gestational diabetes will be examined earlier in the pregnancy, e.g. if there has been gestational diabetes in a previous pregnancy. The test involves having a blood sample taken after having a glucose drink. If this test reveals a suspiciously high blood glucose level, a full glucose tolerance test is done to confirm the diagnosis.

EFFECTS ON THE BABY

Most women with gestational diabetes have completely healthy babies. However, high blood glucose levels can, as described earlier, result in a large baby. If the baby is large, it makes the delivery more difficult; if the baby is too large, an early delivery or a Caesarean section may be necessary. If the mother's blood glucose levels have not been well controlled after the delivery, the baby can have low blood glucose levels.

Since gestational diabetes usually develops in the latter part of pregnancy, after organ formation is complete, congenital defects are not more common than in pregnancies without diabetes.

MANAGEMENT OF GESTATIONAL DIABETES

Many women with gestational diabetes are overweight and gestational diabetes may be controlled with weight control during pregnancy. A full dietary review is necessary: a diet low in fat and with regular spaced meals is recommended. Overweight women should try to minimise weight gain, but should avoid excessive caloric restriction. Usual weight gain during pregnancy is 10–12 kg. Regular exercise is also encouraged, not only for the general wellbeing of the mother, but also to improve the blood glucose control in gestational diabetes.

Despite eating a healthy low-fat diet and exercising regularly, at least one-third of women with gestational diabetes will not have low enough blood glucose levels and will need further treatment. Unfortunately, the tablets used in non-insulin dependent diabetes (NIDDM) are not recommended to be used during pregnancy because they may cause side effects for the baby. Therefore, insulin injections must be used. Usually two even three daily injections are necessary. The amount of insulin needed increases throughout the pregnancy, making it necessary to do regular blood glucose testing at home with frequent dose adjustment. This requires close liaison between the doctor, diabetes educator and the mother-to-be.

Labour and the post-partum period are managed similarly to that described for women with IDDM. Blood glucose levels tend to fall to normal levels immediately after delivery, so that in the majority of cases the diabetes goes away immediately.

LONG-TERM EFFECTS ON INFANT AND MOTHER

A significant number of women with gestational diabetes will develop diabetes (usually NIDDM) later in life. Importantly, the risk of development of diabetes can be reduced by keeping to normal weight and doing regular exercise. Due to the increased risk of developing NIDDM later, regular screening for diabetes is advised (with oral glucose tolerance testing or checks of blood glucose levels), particularly in those women who also have a strong family history of diabetes.

Infants born to women with gestational diabetes will not have diabetes at birth, but they are at increased risk of developing diabetes later in adult life (NIDDM).

Chapter 16

Contraction and Hormone Replacement Therapy

This chapter outlines common methods of contraception and discusses the use of hormone replacement therapy after menopause. It is even more important for women with diabetes to time their pregnancies to occur when they want than it is for women who do not have diabetes.

CONTRACEPTION IN IDDM

Since optimal blood glucose control at conception and during early pregnancy reduces the risk of spontaneous abortions and congenital malformations, contraception advice is a particularly important part of the management of fertile women with insulin dependent diabetes (IDDM). Furthermore, although most women with diabetes can safely have children, some women with severe complications are best advised to decide against pregnancy. The choice between the various methods is largely a matter of patient preference.

Barrier methods (condoms, diaphragms, cervical caps)

Barrier methods are now more popular, largely because of their efficiency in reducing the spread of sexually transmissible diseases. The main problem with this type of method is that there is a moderate failure rate, although this is usually due to incorrect usage. In situations where pregnancy is absolutely contra-indicated, they are not recommended, because of the failure rate. There is no reason for people with diabetes not to use these methods if they find them suitable for their needs.

Oral contraceptive pill

The oral contraceptive pill is a very effective form of contraception for women. In the past, women with IDDM who used the older contraceptive agents containing a higher oestrogen dose and older form of progestogen have needed a higher insulin dose. With the newer preparations, an insulin dosage adjustment is rarely necessary. The new low-dose pills are relatively safe. However, a risk of vein thrombosis exists, and older women who smoke have a higher risk of heart disease with the pill. Oral contraceptive agents should be restricted to young patients without serious diabetic complications or additional vascular risk factors (i.e. smoking, strong family history of ischaemic heart disease) and the newer low-dose agents should always be used.

Intra-uterine devices (IUDs)

Intra-uterine devices (IUDs) are inserted into the uterus and are changed every couple of years. The advantages of the IUD are that they will not affect the blood glucose or lipid levels, and also that the person does not need to regularly consume pills or do anything else in order to avoid becoming pregnant. The main concern is an increased infection risk associated with these devices, which might be a particular concern in patients with poorly controlled diabetes who are more predisposed to developing or continuing infections. IUDs are usually not the first choice of contraceptive agent in women with diabetes, but can be useful in some women.

Sterilisation (tubal ligation)

Tubal ligation, cutting and tying the tubes between the ovaries and the womb, may be advised for women with serious diabetic complications in order to protect from pregnancy. Many women with diabetes request tubal ligation once they have completed their families. It can be done by laparoscopy, which requires only a very small incision.

Vasectomy

Vasectomy means cutting and tying the vas (tube from the testes) in the scrotum of the male partner. Vasectomy may be the method of choice for some couples. This is done under local anaesthetic without admission to hospital.

HORMONE REPLACEMENT THERAPY (HRT)

Hormone replacement therapy (HRT) with oestrogen and progestogen is now recommended for consideration by most post-menopausal women to improve quality of life, and to prevent coronary artery disease and osteoporosis. There are, however, limited data on the use of HRT in women with diabetes, a group at increased risk of coronary artery disease who may theoretically derive even greater benefits from HRT than women who do not have diabetes.

From the limited evidence available, HRT appears to have the same positive effects in lowering cholesterol in women with diabetes as it does in those without. However, in women with diabetes, HRT may increase triglyceride levels. Increased triglyceride levels could have an adverse effect on the arteries and, in rare instances, if very high, could precipitate pancreatitis (inflammation of the pancreas). Thus, blood fat levels, and in particular triglyceride levels, should be checked in women with diabetes while they are using HRT.

The vaginal benefits of replacing oestrogen include cure of vaginal dryness, lessened skin thinning and less tendency to urine infection from thinning of the pelvic floor.

If a woman has had a hysterectomy, only the oestrogen hormone is needed. If the uterus is present, a progesterone hormone is usually added to prevent an increased risk of uterine cancer with oestrogen alone. The hormones are usually taken as tablets, but patches can be worn for absorption through the skin.

For each woman, the individual benefits and risks of HRT should be carefully considered and discussed with her doctor before starting treatment.

Chapter 17

Sexuality and Diabetes

This chapter is an attempt to present an integrated overview of male and female sexuality where one partner has diabetes. By defining sexuality in its broadest terms, I have tried to blend physical, emotional and social issues in an attempt to embrace people as sexual beings.

'Sexuality' can be said to encompass everything one thinks, feels or does during one's life related to being male or female. Therefore, the term encompasses three major areas: the *biological,* the *psychological* and the *social.* The **biological** responses include our male or female bodies, hormones, genitals and the capacity to experience sexual excitement and orgasm, fertility and potential parenthood. The **psychological** responses include body image, perception of one's own appearance and attractiveness to oneself and one's partner (or to potential partners if not in a relationship), and one's ability to engage in sexual activity. The **social** responses include such things as one's communication and relationship with one's partner, and one's sense of integration, affirmation and acceptance in the larger network of family, friends and society.

Sexuality is an intrinsic part of all of us. After all, who of us leaves our sexuality at home when we go shopping or go to work? However, even though it is an intrinsic part of us, how we express ourselves sexually depends on how sexuality was dealt with in our own family, our cultural norms, our religious beliefs, the sex education we received, the sexual experiences we have had, our partner(s) and our ability to communicate about sensitive private thoughts, feelings and needs.

Our society has four main taboo areas: ageing, illness, death and sex. Most people have some degree of discomfort around these areas. We know that only about 10% of Australians have had a really good sexual education.

MYTHS

Because of the 'taboo' about plain speaking about sex, most cultures 'learn' about sexuality via myths spread through the community by sexual jokes, films, books and magazines. Myths float around us and are often so subtly absorbed that we are not aware that we are learning about our own sexuality. Myths have a seductive half-truth to them. For example:

- A real man always wants and is always ready to have sex.
- An erection is essential for sex.
- If you haven't had intercourse or an orgasm, you haven't done it.
- It is the man's job to initiate and orchestrate sex.
- Good sex must be super sex every time.
- Once started, all contact must go on to intercourse and orgasm.
- As you get older, you lose interest in sex and no longer want it.
- Children should not affect your sex life.
- If your partner masturbates, there must be something wrong with you.
- If sex is monotonous, you must not love your partner.
- My partner should be interested in sex when I am.
- If he or she loved me, he or she would automatically know what I like and need during sex and give it to me.

Critically important is the ability to separate and differentiate love, lust and sexual lovemaking ability.

One of my favourite myths is that 'sex is natural'. Think about that! We also believe that 'walking is natural'. Now consider what actually happens: a baby goes through stages of learning then one day, after watching thousands of people around himself or herself walking (demonstrating), the baby takes a step. What happens next? An adult usually cheers and encourages more steps. The baby continues to observe and to practise and gain expertise and mastery. When it comes to sex, we expect to be good at something we have very little real education about (the schoolyard is not an expert source of knowledge). No wonder sexual success is achieved when everything is going OK, and crumbles when ageing, illness or relationship or social stresses come along.

ILLNESS

It is common for people adjusting to any chronic disease to experience sexual and/or relationship difficulties. These can arise as a result of the disease or as a result of the stress, or as a combination of both.

Self-esteem can be affected, especially if already vulnerable. The effect on our self-esteem occurs as our image of ourselves alters with altered body image (such as proneness to infections, weight gain or weight loss, depression, pain), loss of capabilities, changes in social role or changes in status within the family. For men especially, there can be anxiety about change from the strong head of the family to 'the ill one'. There can be treatment and medication side effects generally and sexually.

Very few of us are so confident in our sexuality that when a diagnosis of a chronic condition is made it has no effect on us or our partner. Many people start wondering:
- Is this a good time to stop being sexual?
- Is it safe to be sexual?
- Will changed sexual roles be acceptable?
- Will changed sexual patterns be acceptable to my partner?
- Can I take the risk of exposing myself to my partner?
- How scary is it to be faced with changes?
- How scary is it to not be in control?
- Is it easier simply to stop making love?
- Is it fair to my partner if I start and cannot finish as I used to do before?

Remember the myths mentioned previously? Another message given to us by society is not only that illness removes the capacity for sexual behaviour, but also that it also removes the desire to be sexual.

It is not surprising that self-defeating attitudes and assumptions about sex in general, and about sexual 'performance' and sex roles in particular, can magnify whatever direct effects diabetes may have on sexual desire, arousal, orgasm or activity.

Partners are also affected as they experience anger, guilt, frustration and depression from the changed private and social situations. Lack of knowledge about what is normal and fears about talking to someone about sexuality often prevent people from getting helpful advice.

It is very important to spend some time working out what negative thoughts you have floating around in your head.

- Will my partner still find me attractive?
- Can I still be a good lover?
- Why does it take me so long to get turned on?
- Will my erection last?
- Can I have an orgasm/am I taking too long to have an orgasm?
- How can I have a sex life when I am always so tired?
- Will my partner continue to love me?
- How much should I tell a potential partner and when?
- Can I get pregnant? Can I father a child?
- Will I make my partner feel insecure by suggesting changes to our sexual 'routine'?
- How do I get interested in sex when I am dealing with everything else about having diabetes?
- How can I get people to see me as a sexual person and not only as someone with a condition?
- Am I still a 'man' if I cannot get erections?
- What is my position in the family if I am no longer earning what I used to?

One way to turn these thoughts around is to make a list of the negative thoughts, and then turn them into the positive thoughts you would like to be true. For example:

    I am a lousy lover. ————> I can be a great lover.

Now set about working on how you can achieve this goal, and involve your partner in this shared project (after all, you want it to benefit both of you).

Do not be surprised if you have trouble talking about sex and feelings – you are in the majority. Most of us come from homes where sexuality wasn't discussed, so we have grown up not being practised at this. Remember, there are books, courses and professionals to help you. Be patient, and accept that you are wearing an 'L' plate, i.e. you are a beginner. It can be fun, challenging and ultimately very rewarding.

WHY DO WE MAKE LOVE?

Apart from the obvious biological requirement in procreation, which only takes up a very small percentage of lovemaking frequency, we make love for many reasons.

We make love to show and to receive love and affection, to be reassured of our attractiveness and to reaffirm our masculinity or femininity. We do it for fun, to relieve sexual tension, to relieve non-sexual tension (anger, frustration or sadness), to relieve boredom (say, if there isn't a good movie on TV) or to relieve insomnia. Sometimes we do it because it's expected of us (the media would have us believe that most people do it all the time, last all night, are multi-orgasmic, etc.). Sometimes we do it because our partner wants to or because we think our partner expects it. Sometimes we do it because we need to be hugged and caressed. This is a basic human need. Of course, we also sometimes make love to dominate, hurt or control our partner, or for some sort of gain.

You can see from the above that making love is actually very important for many reasons. If you stop making love, how will those other needs be met? In fact, you can meet all the needs without intercourse, without having an erection and without an orgasm, but not without lovemaking and communication.

SEXUAL RESPONSE CYCLE

There is a basic similarity between the male and female sexual response cycle. One can imagine a journey where first one's senses are triggered to give desire and arousal for sexual activity. This sensual journey may account for about 70% of the cycle and it is in this phase most of the creativity in lovemaking takes place. The body's response builds up in intensity and one enters a phase of desiring more intense stimulation. This period accounts for about 25% of the cycle. The third phase involves either penetration or 'going for the orgasm', and often takes up no more than about 5% of the time. Of course, there are variations on this theme, for example, 'quickies' (orgasms without much mental arousal).

Sensuality 70%	Sexuality 20%	Orgasm I/C 5%

Schematic representation of sexual response cycle

Phase 1: desire
Mental and physical stimulation. Body's information gathering (mental and physical) that it is safe to become aroused.

Phase 2: arousal
Nerve and blood vessel coordination in the pelvis and groin in response to arousal threshold being reached.

Increased blood flow and pelvic congestion resulting in vaginal lubrication or penile erection. Breasts and nipples swell in both men and women. Many women do not find breast stimulation stimulating. The pupils dilate (an erotic signal to the partner). Increases in muscular tension with involuntary pelvic movements. Increased heart rate, blood pressure and breathing.

Phase 3: orgasm
Continued mental and physical stimulation until the orgasmic threshold is reached.

Nerve discharge and muscular contractions resulting in propulsion of ejaculate through the penis, and vaginal and/or uterine contractions, and then relaxation resulting in blood outflow from the penis and the pelvic areas.

Phase 4: resolution
Emotional and physical relaxation. Return to unaroused state.

HOW DIFFICULTIES EXPRESS THEMSELVES IN THESE FOUR PHASES

Desire phase
People can experience sexual desire as anything from a passionate eagerness for sexual contact and arousal to a mild inclination to engage in 'it'. Others experience a seeking of physical closeness, intimacy and connectedness. Desire is expressed by fantasies and thoughts about sex, initiating and responding to sexual overtures, masturbation, reading erotic literature and watching erotic movies.

You will see that *inhibited sexual desire* is at the top of the list for sexual difficulties in the community as it is one of the most common sexual difficulties treated by therapists in the general population. When there is a direct physical basis, it is due to brain injuries, altered hormone production, side effects of medication, poorly controlled blood glucose levels etc. The more common causes are the psychological and relationship difficulties.

The effects of diabetes on sexual desire are probably indirect, arising out of depression, anger, tiredness, fear and effects on relationship and family dynamics. Not all the difficulties may be coming from the person with diabetes. The partner's sexual interest may fall as a result of changes to their feelings, depression, fears, negative thoughts and expectations. Where communication has not been good, the sexual adjustment fragile or the relationship precarious, the added agenda of diabetes can suppress sexual desire.

Arousal phase

It is in this phase that diabetes has the greatest impact in men. By damaging the small blood vessels, it affects the blood flow into the hydraulic system of the penis that causes an erection. Effects on the nerve supply can also affect the mechanism which coordinates the blood flow. The result is an erectile difficulty — a penis not firm enough or lasting long enough for intercourse. As the ability to have erections is so valued in our society, any disturbance to this is bound to have emotional repercussions for the man and his partner. The final difficulty is often a combination of diabetic effects, ageing and psychological effects.

Although there seem to be physiological changes that occur for women with diabetes in the arousal phase, they do not seem to cause sexual difficulties for most of these women. However, thoughts about attractiveness, fears about hypoglycaemia, discomfort from thrush or urinary tract infections, and the same anxieties experienced by men can affect arousal in women.

Performance anxiety is one of the biggest 'headaches' in overcoming sexual difficulties. It can take only one experience of sexual difficulty from any cause for a man or a woman for anxiety to become established. Once thoughts such as 'Will it last this time?', 'I'm taking too long to lubricate.' and 'Am I disappointing my partner?' take hold, they distract from the feelings and sensations that would otherwise occur. Anxiety also causes the release of adrenaline which diverts blood flow away from the genitals to the muscles for 'fight or flight'. There is no survival benefit to being sexually aroused when you are in danger!

Unfortunately, this mechanism interferes with sexual arousal in milder situations as well — the baby crying, someone walking past the bedroom door, a telephone ringing, negative thoughts, etc.

Most men and women have experienced the effects of watching and judging their own sexual performance at some time. This, combined with negative thoughts like 'I can't do it anymore' can block sexual arousal whether there are diabetic effects or not.

Orgasm phase

In men, ejaculation is a two-step process. The first, emission, leads to the release of seminal fluid into the prostatic urethra. The second phase, ejaculation, involves contraction of the muscles in the penis and the pelvic floor, resulting in release of the fluid to the outside. The muscles at the neck of the bladder are contracted so that the fluid is expelled to the outside rather than back into the bladder.

The expulsive contractions in men are equivalent to the muscular contractions in the outer third of the vagina and the uterus in women during orgasm.

When the nerves to the genital area are affected, it is possible for men to have dry orgasms (no ejaculation), decreased intensity of orgasm, inability to reach orgasm, or ejaculation with an absence of any feeling of orgasm. In women, there are weak, altered or absent orgasms.

SEXUAL DIFFICULTIES

All sexual difficulties are caused by some combination of:
1. ignorance;
2. unrealistic expectations;
3. performance anxiety or general anxiety;
4. poor relationship and communication skills; and
5. medical causes.

Range of sexual difficulties experienced in the community

MEN

(a) Desire difficulties
(b) Erectile difficulties
(c) Ejaculatory difficulties
(d) Altered orgasm sensations

WOMEN

(a) Desire difficulties
(b) Orgasm difficulties
(c) Dyspareunia (pain on intercourse)
(d) Vaginismus (spasm of the muscles around the vagina)
(e) Altered orgasm sensations

Having diabetes does not exempt you from any of these sexual difficulties, but neither does diabetes create any difficulties not experienced by the some people with other medical problems. As diabetes can affect nerves and blood vessels, we would expect there to be sexual consequences as the regulation of blood flow and nerve coordination to the genitals is affected.

SEXUAL RESPONSE CHANGES FOR WOMEN WITH DIABETES

Interestingly, relatively few studies have been carried out to evaluate the effect of diabetes on female sexuality. A review of 11 studies in 1993 evaluated the prevalence of sexual dysfunction in diabetic females. The results indicated that diabetic women experienced low sexual desire, orgasm difficulties and painful intercourse, although not significantly more than women in the general population. In some studies there were more arousal difficulties than in non-diabetic women. Neuropathy, microvascular and macrovascular disease, duration of diabetes and glucose control were not predictive of sexual difficulties. However, psychosocial factors such as disease acceptance, relationship adjustment and depression were correlated with sexual difficulties.

This confirms our own study at St Vincent's Hospital Diabetes Centre carried out in 1989. We found that a woman's sexual satisfaction related to her pre-diabetes sexual history and relationship happiness, rather than to any particular problems arising from the diabetes.

A study carried out in the USA in 1993 by Wincze demonstrated that women with diabetes did have significantly less physiological arousal (lubrication and vaginal changes). However, these women did not report more sexual difficulties. Psychosocial factors are undoubtedly critically important in female sexual happiness.

SEXUAL RESPONSE CHANGES FOR MEN WITH DIABETES

By comparison, the sexual difficulties of men with diabetes have been extensively studied. They report decreases in sexual desire and arousal and erectile difficulties (attaining an erection sufficient for penetration or keeping an erection for sufficient time). Studies have indicated that erectile difficulties are between two and five times more common in diabetic men than in non-diabetic men. Diabetes is probably the single most common cause of erectile difficulties. About 35–55% of men with diabetes have erectile difficulties at some time. The incidence of erectile difficulties increases with age at the same relative rate as in the general population.

The onset of the erectile difficulties is often gradual, with increasing difficulty in obtaining and maintaining an erection. The erection gradually becomes less firm and of diminished duration. However, orgasms are definitely possible, although the feeling of orgasm is altered. Retrograde ejaculation (ejaculation into the bladder) can also occur.

Reversible erectile difficulty can also occur with poor diabetic control, either at first presentation of the disease or during the illness.

AGE-RELATED SEXUAL CHANGES

It is important to understand what happens to all of us as we mature so that fear and unrealistic expectations do not rob us of our sexual potential. Care needs to be taken to separate normal age-related changes that happen to everyone from specific diabetes-related difficulties.

MEN

(a) Take longer to achieve an erection.
(b) Erections not as firm.
(c) Take longer to ejaculate.
(d) Orgasmic contractions less forceful.
(e) Greater droop.
(f) Decrease in automatic functioning, i.e. OK after a nap, but not after busy day.

(g) Increased latency time, i.e. increased time between ability to get erections.
(h) Decreased genital sensitivity.

WOMEN
(a) Decreased lubrication.
(b) Increased tightness and sensitivity of the vagina.
(c) Dyspareunia (painful intercourse due to causes like prolapses, constipation, urethral irritation etc.)
(d) Decreased force of orgasmic contractions.
(e) Painful uterine contractions.
(f) Decreased genital sensitivity.

Research shows that the most important factors for older people to have a satisfying and enjoyable sex life are positive attitudes and expectations, and an enthusiastic partner. Sex may be physically different, but this does not mean that it cannot be satisfying, enjoyable and fun.

COMMUNICATING ABOUT SEX

As mentioned earlier, most of us have not been brought up in homes where intimate problems and sexuality were openly discussed. Therefore, talking about sex can be threatening, especially if we fear rejection or ridicule, or an increase in tension in an already stressed relationship.

Common issues to discuss in sexual relationships include: frequency and types of sexual activity, new sexual activities, use of fantasy, desire for more intimacy, desire for greater spontaneity, less specific role expectations, reduced focus on intercourse and orgasm, more non-sexual touching, more tenderness and gentleness, more assertiveness and passion, not being taken for granted, more open communication about any of the above, and reassurance that you are loved and needed.

DEALING WITH SEXUAL PROBLEMS

Most of the sexual difficulties experienced by people with diabetes can be helped through education. Information is needed on how to enhance sexuality, improve communication, decrease stereotypical sexual behaviourial expectations, practise pleasurable sexual behaviours and avoid non-pleasurable ones. People need to look at practical ways to improve overall happiness, and should seek professional help earlier rather than later. It is important to put embarrassment and pride aside and use what is available in the community.

CONDITIONS FOR BETTER SEX

We all have our own 'good conditions' for sex and, if we are to be happy with our sex lives, it is critically important that we know what these conditions are and strive to meet them.

1. Adequate liking and acceptance of yourself. Sense of being entitled to good sex.
2. Reasonable physical and emotional fitness.
3. Reasonable energy.
4. Emotional availability for sex.
5. Some degree of pleasurable anticipation.
6. Reasonable confidence in your sexual performance.
7. Some attraction to your partner.
8. Reasonable communication/intimacy/trust between you and your partner.
9. Reasonably secure, private and comfortable environment.
10. Adequate sexual knowledge/skill.

WHAT YOU CAN EXPECT ONCE PROFESSIONAL HELP IS SOUGHT?

1. Full medical history, examination and relevant tests.
2. Full sexual history, examination and relevant tests.
3. Education about normal sexuality and sexual enhancement techniques, age-related normal changes, diabetes-related sexual changes.
4. Individual psychological help.
5. Relationship enhancement.
6. Medication.
7. Non-invasive sexual aids.
8. Surgery.

SPECIFIC SEXUAL DIFFICULTIES: THERAPY

Inhibited sexual desire in men and women

This is the most common, complex and difficult sexual difficulty to treat. To overcome it requires the commitment and patience of both partners and their therapist. Usually the problem has been gradual in onset, with acknowledgment of the difficulty finally coming following a trauma such as the diagnosis of diabetes or threat of divorce.

Classically, it is the lower drive partner who is complained about and brought for therapy. Inhibited sexual desire has to be differentiated from sexual phobias, normal low sex drive, normal and appropriate inhibition of sexual desire, depression and low sexual desire due to hormonal states and medication.

The person with a normal low sex drive will lack erotic fantasies or interest in any sexual activity. They will rarely be moved to seek any form of sexual release. The secondary form of lowered sex desire is more common. Here the person experiences desire, but only under certain conditions. Both men and women may masturbate to climax at regular frequency, may have sex with other partners or may need very specific conditions, e.g. special clothing, but will have no interest in sexual activity with their regular partner. Sexual desire is particularly absent when and with whom our society designates that it would be most appropriate to experience it. More women present as the lower sex drive partner because women do not have the testosterone boost (men's testosterone levels are 20–30 times higher than women's). This means that women are more sensitive to the inhibitors mentioned below.

Inhibitors of sexual interest and response

1. Lack of time
2. Fatigue
3. Physical discomfort
4. Lack of emotional wellbeing — guilt, frustration, anger, resentment, worry, sadness, depression, shame
5. Lack of pleasurable anticipation
6. Lack of attraction to partner
7. Performance anxiety — trying too hard
8. Poor self-esteem/poor sexual self-esteem
9. Unhelpful thoughts — distractions

10. Inadequate mental and sensual stimulation
11. Inadequate physical environment
12. Recreational drugs, alcohol, sedatives, medications
13. Poor sex education
14. Negative sexual attitudes
15. Lack of non-demand affection and companionship — fun
16. Lack of trust — fidelity issues, unresolved jealousy
17. Insecurity — lack of commitment
18. Poor communication
19. Lack of intimacy
20. Lack of respect
21. Lack of enhancers
    Female: closeness, intimacy, affection, non-sexual contact, romance
    Male: erotica, nudity, magazines, movies, varied lovemaking, lingerie
22. Tension in the relationship — conflict: money, independence, decision making, status in family, duties in family
23. Pursuer/distancer — relationship difficulty
24. Partner response

Medical intervention is only necessary if there are hormonal imbalances in testosterone (or prolactin or thyroxine). Low testosterone is not common in men and no long-term sexual benefits occur with giving a normal man testosterone. Adding testosterone to HRT in menopausal women can aid sexual interest and responsiveness where a low free serum testosterone has been measured. Anti-depressants have an appropriate role where depression is a factor. Dietary supplements occasionally help in energy levels.

Most therapy centres on individual and couples issues being resolved, along with romance and lovemaking skills being added.

Male

Erectile difficulties

Erectile difficulties can be caused by psychological problems, relationship difficulties, poor sexual techniques and medical problems. It is almost impossible to have a medically caused erectile difficulty without some personal and relationship difficulty.

If you think back to the reasons we make love, you will come to the conclusion that most are possible without an erection. When counselling helps to remove the individual's or couple's barriers to creative sexuality, and improves intimacy, erectile difficulties often improve. In medically caused erectile difficulties, counselling alone cannot provide erections. Some will choose to accept this situation and elect not to pursue further options. Penetrative sex is not everything in either lovemaking or life enjoyment.

However, many people have always enjoyed penetrative sex and want to be able to continue enjoying it. Here are some options.

Mechanical devices for erectile difficulties

1. Penile splint (supports a soft penis to allow penetration and ejaculation in the vagina).
2. Constriction ring (rubber rings to prevent the outflow of blood from the penis).
3. Vacuum devices (create negative pressure around the penis so that blood flows into the penis and is then trapped by a rubber band).
4. Intracavernosal vasodilators (injection into the shaft of the penis of Prostaglandin E1, papaverine, phentolamine or combinations of these three to produce an erection. Prostaglandin E1 is most commonly used).
5. Intrapenile prostheses (two rods inserted into the penis to give either a permanent erection or an inflatable one).
6. Revascularisation surgery (improving the blood supply to the penis).
7. Venous ligation surgery (closing of veins where there is an outflow problem which causes a too quick loss of erection).

The partner should be fully involved in all the discussions. There is no point in investing in an option which your partner does not want to use.

Ejaculatory difficulties

Humankind seems to be the only species that values 'lasting' in intercourse and, even then, this seems to be a more recent development — perhaps due to the sexual revolution. For all other species, it seems to be 'on and off' as quickly as it is possible to get the job (impregnation) done.

Premature ejaculation (PE) is the most common male sexual difficulty, affecting up to a third of the male population. PE is defined as a persistent lack of voluntary control over ejaculation.

It is important to keep in mind that we are not all born equal, e.g. not all us of us can run a 3-minute mile. Some people are born with intuitive sensitivity to themselves and their partner, some are born with very little interest in sex and quite simply are always going to find it hard going. The rest of us are somewhere in the middle with mixed talents which can improve with education and practice. Do not forget the example about learning to walk, because in good sex we have to learn not only to be in control of ourselves, but to coordinate with another separate individual.

Men with PE progress very quickly from excitement to orgasm, and the orgasm is often experienced as only mildly pleasurable. Anxiety plays an important role because almost all sufferers have good ejaculatory control during solitary masturbation.

Management options

1. Accommodation of the PE into the lovemaking style of the couple, for example, the other partner has an orgasm by oral or manual stimulation either before or after intercourse. Many women will not have an orgasm through intercourse no matter how long the man is able to last. Many men are able to last longer in the second round of lovemaking and this is an option with younger men who can have another erection within a reasonable time of ejaculating.
2. Sex therapy: sex education with counselling about special techniques.
3. Medication. The SSRI drugs (Prozac and Zoloft), used in the treatment of depression, delay orgasm and can be very useful in quickly reversing a distressing situation. The gains seem to remain after the medication is stopped.

Retrograde/dry ejaculation

This is relatively common in older men. It can be caused by the ejaculate going back into the bladder or a failure of secretions to collect in the urethra from which they are ejaculated. The most common causes are prostate operations and diabetic autonomic neuropathies (nerve damage).

Retrograde ejaculation can often be surgically corrected. However, many men chose not to worry about it once they understand what is happening. Lovemaking can be fully enjoyed except that there is no 'mess' and the sensation of orgasm can be a little different. If pregnancy is desired, the sperm can be retrieved from the post-masturbation urine and artificially inseminated.

Inhibited/retarded ejaculation

This is mostly a psychogenic problem (although some medications can cause this problem), where there is recurrent and persistent inhibition of orgasm. This can range in severity from never having ejaculated by masturbation alone to never having ejaculated in the vagina. The most common variant is that the man is unable to ejaculate in the vagina, but can masturbate to orgasm with the partner. Many psychological factors may be responsible, including fear of impregnating the partner, religious beliefs, guilt, hostility towards the partner, oedipal fears of retaliation and fears of defiling the partner with semen. Counselling (often long-term and intensive) is the required treatment.

Painful ejaculation

This difficulty can have a psychogenic basis, but acute genito-urinary infection and anatomical problems have to be excluded first.

Women

Orgasmic difficulties: therapy

In the biology versus sexual fun stakes, orgasmic ease for women is a fairly late evolutionary development not necessary for human survival. As far as we know, primate (monkey) females do not have orgasms.

In cultures where women are not encouraged to know their bodies and explore how they work — and where they are also taught that only sexuality with the husband after legal marriage is acceptable — there are higher rates of sexual difficulties, including difficulty reaching orgasm.

Once a woman knows how to reach orgasm herself, she is in a much better position to show her partner. A man cannot make a woman have an orgasm, he can only help. There are very few conditions that prevent a woman from reaching orgasm if she is getting the kind of stimulation she needs for long enough.

Conditions where the nerve supply to the genital area is lost or where sexual centres in the brain are damaged obviously affect the ability to orgasm. All other difficulties arise from personal, social, relationship and technical causes. Even women with clitoroidectomies (surgical removal of the clitoris) can have orgasms, if they receive enough stimulation mentally and to the nerves running along the pelvic rim.

In diabetes, secondary loss of orgasmic ability can occur with poor diabetic control, urinary tract infections, thrush, depression, relationship difficulties and tiredness. Occasionally, it takes one episode of painful or forced sex for a difficulty to develop.

It is important to remember that only about 30% of women climax with intercourse only and about 30% of women have never climaxed with a partner.

In overcoming orgasmic difficulties, there has to be an understanding of the particular woman's history. She then needs to be educated about becoming friends with her body – to understand her conditions for good sex, to be able to communicate her needs to her partner and then to have patience to practise because it can take up to 60 minutes to reach orgasm when first learning or relearning.

Dyspareunia

This occurs when a woman experiences pain with intercourse. It may always have been the case, may come on after a period of normal sexual function, or may occur only in certain situations. The commonest cause in all cases is inadequate arousal. Medical causes need to be excluded, especially vaginitis (usually caused by thrush), pelvic inflammatory disease and pelvic congestion syndrome.

Vaginismus

Vaginismus occurs when there is an involuntary spasm of the pelvic floor muscles in response to pressure/touch at the vaginal entrance or anticipation of vaginal penetration by tampon, speculum, finger or penis.

Usually, there is some history of a repressive upbringing with shame around sexuality. The sex education is usually very poor with distorted ideas about anatomy. This can lead to fears of being too small, of being ripped or hurt. There may be some childhood trauma, but it may not be overt sexual abuse. Fear of emotional or physical abuse at the hands of a more powerful male, or of being taken over, can lead to a need to maintain strong boundaries – to the point where penetration is felt to be intrusive or invasive. Vaginismus can also develop secondary to a precipitating event like a painful delivery, vaginal infection or sexual assault.

A starting point in overcoming this sexual difficulty is understanding the history and situation, and working through the blocks. Sex education, relaxation exercises, pelvic muscle exercises, lots of body work and relationship work are vital. Time and patience are essential.

Many women with vaginismus are orgasmic with manual and oral stimulation, and enjoy lovemaking if penetration is not attempted.

Chapter 18

Diabetes and Stress Management

THE STRESS REACTION AND ITS EFFECT

Differences between short and long-term stress

Have you ever experienced a near miss in a car or been involved in a heated argument? These are good examples of short-term stress. How did you feel? Did you breath faster? Was your heart pounding? Did you have butterflies in your stomach? Were you sweating? Did your muscles tense up?

These symtoms occur very quickly and are caused by stress hormones. These hormones (also called counter-regulatory hormones) include glucagon, adrenaline, growth hormone and cortisol, (*see* Chapter 1, 'What is diabetes?'). Apart from the stress symptoms described, **their net effect is to raise blood glucose levels.** This effect is somewhat controversial. As you might appreciate, it is hard to measure scientifically as it is ethically tricky to place real people in real situations of stress and then test their blood sugars. The sudden, unexpected bursts of stress in experiments don't seem to change blood sugars too much, but people vary a lot. Longer-term stress or anxiety, unresolved problems or even the one hundred and one brief stresses in a busy day may be more of a problem to overall blood glucose patterns. Work pressures, dealing with others, finances, relationships, exams, etc are not exactly life-threatening, but the way they are managed does affect our physical and emotional wellbeing. Our capacity to dwell on the overall meaning of these experiences and consider their future impact can also generate a 'stress reaction'.

I can't tell you exactly how much stress will cause what rise in blood glucose, but you need to look at how your particular stress relates to your overall pattern of blood glucose levels. (This is independent of your food, exercise, medication and any illness).

Longer term stress is, of course, harder to pinpoint compared to short-term stress. It is as if we are accumulating stress points and the body's reaction is not as dramatic. The symptoms are more likely to be those of withdrawal (depression), loss of interest in general, vague headaches, poor sleep, irritability, eating more (usually, but some eat less) and being less active. If these signs persist, quality of health and life will suffer.

As well as the above physical symptoms, emotional reactions also come into play. In the short term, shock, anger and denial in response to a crisis may be quite reasonable ways of coping, but if maintained over the longer term they do not fit well with the permanent task of having to handle diabetes.

So far, then, the picture can be summarised as follows. *Stress, in the short or long term, has the potential to:*

1. raise blood glucose levels;
2. increase blood pressure;
3. indirectly lead to unhealthy behaviours (e.g. eating badly, being less active);
4. generate negative emotions; and
5. impair our capacity to think clearly or make good judgments.

Being 'stressed' is in itself a stress, so all of this is a sort of vicious circle which can be difficult to break. There are, of course, many things concerning diabetes about which you need to be 'worried'. Rather than remaining worried, let us consider how to move from a situation of 'naturally worried' to that of 'confident concern'. (There is evidence in psychological literature that those who can see the inherent dangers in a situation cope better compared to those who 'do not worry about it', i.e. deny it. The former group is more likely to keep to their management tactics most of the time and this, in turn, is more likely to head off any long-term body damage.)

SOME PRINCIPLES OF STRESS MANAGEMENT

The key word here is *management*. No one can avoid being 'stressed' at times. In fact, it has long been recognised that a certain degree of stress is an effective motivation as it helps us concentrate or focus on a particular problem or situation. A good example of this is if we are ever asked to perform in some way to an audience. The worst fear here would be to clam up altogether and make a fool of yourself. If this fear takes over and becomes too great, the chances of actually doing just that increase dramatically. If the tension can be kept to a manageable level, we are able to concentrate on the task and are probably helped by the fact that smaller amounts of tension prior to the performance have led us to actually study, prepare and rehearse the situation. Interestingly enough, being completely relaxed may not help things either.

It is important to realise that stress management is not the same as stress elimination. I have seen many people over the years feel they are some sort of failure or cannot cope because the 'stress' still remains. Why are you a failure if the diabetes will not go away? What if it is your family that is causing the stress? How easy is it to change jobs in these economic times? The elimination–solution approach in these situations is not going to work.

Two messages arise from this:
- Stress management, if effective, can stop negative feelings and thoughts from reaching 'paralysing' levels or reduce stress to a level where one can function more effectively.
- Stress itself is not necessarily the problem – the problem may be one's attitude towards the stress-producing situation.

Here are some suggestions to start the management approach.

1. Consider the source or cause of the stress

Surprisingly, this is harder to do than it looks and most people have different 'problems'. Some are directly in front of us, while others are sort of in the background quietly fermenting away. (I am not forgetting diabetes as a stress, but life's problems can muck up the diabetes and diabetes can interfere in everyday living.) In trying to regain some sort of balance, the next step is...

2. Ask yourself what do you actually want or need

This requires a fairly realistic appraisal of your overall situation and one of the needs may often be a bit of help from others. This social support, either from family, friends or colleagues, is an important aide to overall coping. It also gives those closer to you a role in your management. Examples could be how you prefer to be helped (if ever!) if you get caught with a hypo, or how your food pattern fits in with your family's. This communication of needs is in itself a useful stress reduction skill. It can also help sort out real priorities.

3. Consider what CAN and what CANNOT be changed

This sort of analysis often leads to the realisation that most things can be modified. Maybe things are not as rigid as you thought or were lead to believe. It may be a bit risky, but have the courage to try different approaches. Most things in diabetes management are not set in concrete. If something does not work too well, negotiate and explore alternatives. Your medical advisers are there to help you help yourself – you are not there to please them.

4. Consider how you manage your time, assert your needs and communicate in general

These are what I would call the nuts and bolts of stress management style courses. They are useful life skills for everyone. If successful, they can free up more time and energy for getting on with what you choose to do rather than being bogged down by what you are forced to do. They could take up another chapter to elaborate fully, but most major hospitals have access to these types of courses, run by appropriately trained people. (Indeed, the NSW Department of Health recommends stress management courses — typically 6–8 weeks.) Being aware of community resources is also a good stress buffer.

5. Do not build in failure

This is a special risk early on in the 'unwanted' career. Health advisers of all types can often inadvertently convey the message that the only way to avoid diabetes' black holes is to do everything suggested all of the time. The only non-negotiable thing is that we all need some insulin. Food, exercise and monitoring blood glucose patterns are not inflexible and scientific knowledge is changing all the time. For example, following set diets for weight loss probably does not work over the long term and could be unhealthy. Ten years ago, to suggest that sugar as part of a meal would not necessarily compromise control would have been some sort of dietary heresy! In other words, you can do most of the things suggested most of the time, but not all of the things all of the time and that's OK.

If, however, after an honest appraisal of your lifestyle, changes need to be made, do not try and do everything at once — it may be too stressful and carries a high risk of failure. Take things one at a time and be proud of what you do achieve.

Consider the 3 R's: *rest, relaxation and recreation*. The principle here is that, in order to be able to cope with everything, we need to be in reasonable 'shape', physically and emotionally, ourselves. I do not mean super-fit in an athletic sense, but being as 'strong' as possible for ourselves. Worrying (even if there are real reasons to do so) can only go so far. One of the problems with diabetes is that it is a 'back-to-front' condition, i.e. its management and a lot of time and effort are constantly devoted to avoiding body problems that have not yet happened. This is in contrast to most other medical complaints that just happen and usually get fixed. This preventive approach demands a 'selfish' response. If you are feeling OK with you, then you are freer to deal with others. Rest and recreational activities that you enjoy provide a sort of 'time out' as well as having healthy side effects.

These suggestions are only meant to be a starting point if stress reaches a level where your capacity to cope is pushed too far. A further chapter could probably examine attitudes and how they affect the way we think, and vice versa. There are probably hundreds of examples of how a particular belief or attitude can lead to higher stress, but consider the following as an example. All of us like to achieve a good result if we are measured physically, whether it be weight, cholesterol, blood pressure etc. It may be that when testing your blood glucose level, your anxiety may increase prior to the actual reading on the machine. Psychologically, if the reading is out of range or unexpected, it is as if the machine is making some sort of moral judgment — 'You've been naughty!', or 'You've failed again!' or 'The diabetes is winning!' This can cause anxiety or guilt so that each testing time is associated with stress (apart from the holes in the fingers!). Testing then could be learned to emphasise only negative aspects. This has been called *learned helplessness*.

Can we replace this with *learned optimism* (not wishful thinking, but confidence based on solid results)? I think so. It is *not* easy and requires a bit of talking to yourself, but in this example it might be possible to see that testing is a window to the inside, providing useful information as a stepping stone for action. The attitude shift could be: 'this is the best, most accurate way for me to know what I need to know to enable me to run this part of my life...I might not always like what I see, but it is better than not knowing at all. If my overall pattern is going OK, I don't have to do it to excess.' As I previously said, it is not always easy, but most of us are not as trapped as we might think.

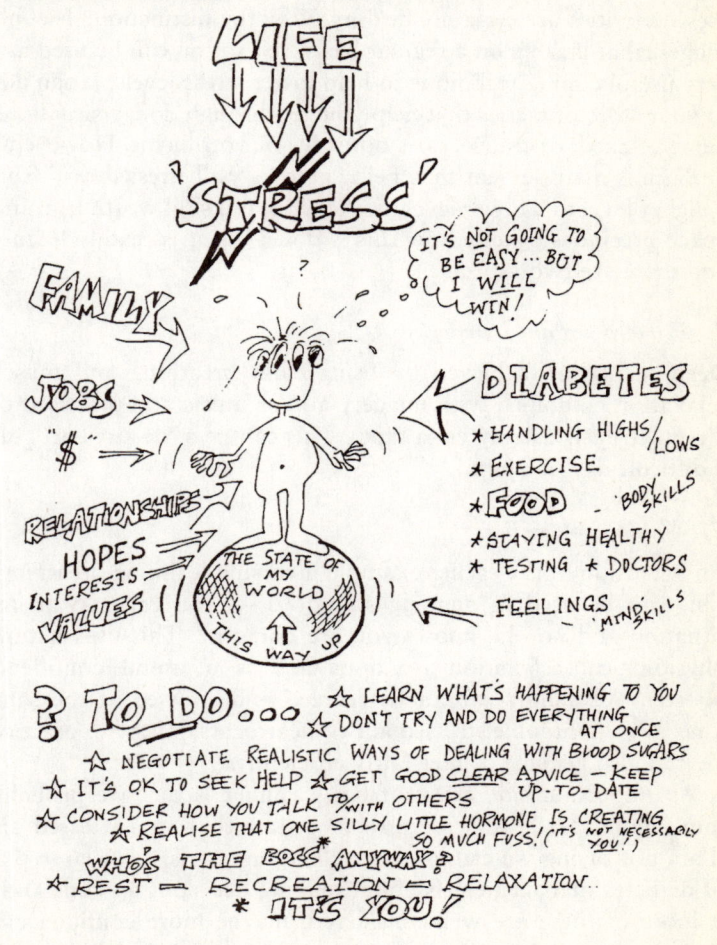

[Hand-drawn illustration: "LIFE" with arrows pointing down to "STRESS" (in lightning-bolt style). A figure stands on a globe labeled "THE STATE OF MY WORLD — THIS WAY UP", thinking "IT'S NOT GOING TO BE EASY...BUT I WILL WIN!". Arrows point in from "FAMILY", "JOBS", "$", "RELATIONSHIPS", "HOPES", "INTERESTS", "VALUES". On the right: "DIABETES — ★ HANDLING HIGHS/LOWS ★ EXERCISE ★ FOOD — BODY SKILLS ★ STAYING HEALTHY ★ TESTING ★ DOCTORS — FEELINGS — MIND SKILLS".

*Below: "? TO DO ooo
★ LEARN WHAT'S HAPPENING TO YOU
★ DON'T TRY AND DO EVERYTHING AT ONCE
★ NEGOTIATE REALISTIC WAYS OF DEALING WITH BLOOD SUGARS
★ IT'S OK TO SEEK HELP ★ GET GOOD CLEAR ADVICE — KEEP UP-TO-DATE
★ CONSIDER HOW YOU TALK TO/WITH OTHERS
★ REALISE THAT ONE SILLY LITTLE HORMONE IS CREATING SO MUCH FUSS! (IT'S NOT NECESSARILY YOU!)
WHO'S THE BOSS ANYWAY?
★ REST = RECREATION = RELAXATION...
★ IT'S YOU!"]*

THE ROLE OF RELAXATION

I would recommend that everyone devotes some time, say once a week or once a fortnight, to 'formal' relaxation. For the reasons given about the stress reaction, I would certainly recommend this for people with diabetes. By 'formal' relaxation I mean spending, say, half an hour or so *specifically* devoted to achieving a fairly deeply relaxed state. We all have many ways of 'informal' relaxation — e.g. sitting in a hot bath, reading, hobbies, visiting friends, visiting interesting places or listening to music. Relaxation is a side effect of doing these things, but not the sole purpose, and these activities are certainly healthy. Why the distinction? I would suggest that if done on a regular basis, relaxation can be used as a very useful coping technique to help lower stress levels. It can add to your store of tactics that help you get through dodgy situations. Being relaxed, of course, does not solve our problems. However, if our aim is management then being able to 'pull stress down' from a higher level to a lower level (not to zero) is a skill worth learning. Space precludes exactly how this is done, but it is readily learned and there are two aspects.

1. *Formal training/practice*

Deep relaxation achieved by using calm breathing and muscle relaxation combined with imagery and/or music and practised on a regular basis usually via a tape. (This can be a 'de-stresser' after a difficult day or upset.)

2. *Waking relaxation*

An extension of the earlier example involving 'calming breathing'. This can be used in ongoing situations — you can stay in the situation and no one knows you are doing it. This uses natural physiological relaxation reactions and is a useful confidence booster. We simply cannot be relaxed and stressed at the same time. We can become stressed in two heartbeats, but, with practice, we can also become calmer fairly efficiently.

An important side effect of being calmer is that we probably think more clearly in a more relaxed state than in a stressed one (I am not saying we cannot think clearly in a crisis). A large part of diabetes management is about making decisions — constantly. If more of these are well-considered, maybe more confidence in their outcome follows, freeing up time to grapple with all the other realities of life and resulting in a greater sense of control.

A CONCLUDING PLAN

Diabetes involves the following considerations. If these issues are successfully tackled, a lot of the stress is balanced.

1. **What are the aims of your overall treatment?**
   What is realistic for you? Do not build in guilt.
   What can you actually do given your circumstances? Be honest.
2. **Be aware that it is not easy but still mostly do-able.**
   It is never too late.
3. **You will get fed up from time to time.**
4. **Exercise.**
   This is probably an underrated, but very important feature of stress management. (Do not get stressed about this! Simply become more active – even gentle walking helps.)
5. **Learn relaxation.**
   Adopt relaxation techniques with which you are comfortable.

Diabetes is complicated. Stay up to date and deal with caring health professionals you can trust. It's good to know how your body works so you know why you are asked to do all this stuff. Diabetes educators don't bite and there is no loss of face in asking for help.

In summary, if something as difficult as diabetes can be felt to be reasonably managed then the lift to self-esteem can do wonders for handling the rest of life's inevitable stress.

Chapter 19

The Adolescent Years

This chapter reviews some of the problems of having diabetes during adolescence — and gives hints for making it an easier time for the whole family.

Adolescence! The mere word conjures up images of awkwardness, self-consciousness, rebellion and peer pressure, along with hormonal and physical upheaval. Having diabetes adds yet a further challenge throughout this time, and often leads to a deterioration in metabolic control.

There is no 'typical' adolescent, but usually there is a set of typical changes which are occurring which impact on their lives and their families, such as searching for independence, finding an identity and pulling away from the family. Having to cope with diabetes adds to these demands. Despite all the recent information on the benefits of good metabolic control, adhering to a regimen of diet regulation, glucose testing and daily insulin injections becomes a difficult task for an adolescent. Non-adherence to this usually becomes the main problem. Combined with this, there are the physical and hormonal changes which also tend to upset the glucose control.

To the onlooker, health care workers, parents and doctors, it often appears so simple: what the adolescent needs to do is to manage their diabetes by testing regularly and making appropriate insulin adjustments. However, the reality is that nothing can make them become more responsible for their diabetes during this time until they understand the need for good control, want that control and feel capable of achieving it.

Some parents find that the only thing to do is to just sit back and wait for the adolescent period to end. It always does and the emerging adult is sometimes scarcely recognisable as the rebellious, difficult teenager of the past.

GETTING PHYSICAL

Physical and hormonal changes occurring during this intense period of time can also lead to a rise in glucose levels. Often this is due to increased insulin resistance, which requires increases in the insulin dose. These may need to be made every few weeks, which may require contact with the endocrinologist or diabetes educator. Especially for girls, this may be a time of weight gain as their body takes on the female form. Combined with more insulin (due to the resistance), this may lead to even more weight gain. Careful monitoring is required as this may be the time when shots are missed and poor eating habits occur in the vain attempt to control or lose weight.

Adolescents are not always aware that the changes which are occurring to their body during puberty can also upset their glucose control. All they feel is that the whole diabetes thing is getting too difficult and they just give up. Explaining these changes to them and offering sympathetic support may help them understand why insulin doses have to be altered and why their blood glucose fluctuates, sometimes without obvious reason.

DARING TO BE DIFFERENT

During adolescence, the pressure to fit in and be like everyone else becomes very real. It is a time when having an adequate self-image helps an adolescent feel accepted as an individual. Friends become one of the main focus points of their lives, which is reflected in doing the same things, playing the same music, wearing the same clothes, eating the same food and watching the same movies as their friends. They start to worry a lot about their appearance and not much about anything else.

Having diabetes can interfere with this lifestyle, as it can with any age group, and it makes them appear different. Diabetes does impose certain restrictions on a person's life and routines, and can make that person feel as if they stand out in the crowd. Thus, these restrictions are the first to go out the window. Issues such as long-term complications do not even come into an adolescent's picture of him/herself at this point, most think they are invincible or immortal. In fact, we all find it hard to restrict ourselves today to avoid something in 10–20 years' time.

Here are some ways that having diabetes can make an adolescent appear different.

1. having a hypo in front of friends;
2. not being able to eat excessive amounts of junk food;
3. having to inject insulin in front of friends;
4. more frequent visits to the doctor — being labelled as 'sickly';
5. having to have meals on or near to time on a daily basis;
6. having restrictions placed upon them by parents, e.g. not staying over at a friends house or not going camping for the weekend;
7. doing blood glucose readings; and
8. having bruises on their stomach (girls especially) or legs from injections, which show up more in summer when playing sport.

This desire not to be seen as different can show itself in the form of what is termed by parents and health professionals as 'mismanagement' behaviours. Behaviours such as missed shots, false test results, not bothering to do any tests, taking extra insulin to cover extra food eaten, eating inappropriate food and poor injection technique are common in adolescence. These behaviours are an attempt to indicate that they are just like everyone else, but are often the factors which result in poor glycaemic control.

SOME HELPFUL HINTS

While the problems influencing treatment adherence spring primarily from being an adolescent, each person should be assessed as an individual and not lumped into the too-hard adolescent basket.

While some parents find it best just to sit this adolescent period out, there are tips that parents can consider to help the adolescent through this time. Each person needs to have his or her problems heard with a kind ear and a sympathetic manner. Try, as hard as it may be, to understand the teenager's point of view without immediate censure.

As the adolescent strives for more independence, it is also the time when parents and health care personnel tend to expect adolescents to take a more active role in their diabetes management. They supervise them less, but often without providing enough information and skills to manage their diabetes. It is possible that gradually handing over care to them before adolescence has taken full hold, and before non-diabetic priorities start to compete, may help them see the benefit of good diabetes management for themselves.

It is good to set some limits — being firm about major issues of care and being flexible about other, less important ones. If possible, they should go and see the health care provider by themselves, so they may feel free to discuss problems or frustrations without parents present.

Communication pathways often tend to fade during this time, and parents start to feel alienated from their child. Conversations start to become mechanistic rather than holistic, and parents, in an attempt to still feel as though they have some control over their adolescent with diabetes, often just ask what the blood glucose levels have been because the adolescent will not divulge how they are. This can leave the adolescent feeling like he or she is just a blood glucose reading to the parent rather than a person. Of course, if these levels are continually high, this only increases the adolescent's avoidance of doing self blood glucose monitoring or leads to figures being made up to pacify the parent.

Sexuality, alcohol and employment are potential problems that start to become a concern for a young person. These factors play a role in any teenager's life, but also need to be addressed by the adolescent with diabetes. There could be potential problems, such as hypos with alcohol or at work, or disclosing information about diabetes to employers (*see* chapters 11, 'Hypoglycaemia' and 22, 'Who should be told?'). Good communication lines need to be open if these issues are to be discussed freely. Counselling help is available if it is needed; some diabetes centres have psychologists attached or have access to outside therapists.

It is often the case that the parents, the health care personnel and the adolescent all have different expectations about what is acceptable diabetes control and good diabetes management. Diabetes needs to be fitted in to the lifestyle of the adolescent for acceptable diabetes management to occur, not the other way around. Everyone involved should have a clear agreement as to what is going to be a reasonable level of control throughout this time. Having these expectations discussed as a team, i.e. patient, doctor, parent and dietitian, will allow everyone concerned to have a say. Be patient and do not expect perfection. Priorities change during adolescence. They often forget to do lots of other things as well, so parents should not expect regular blood glucose readings when nothing else is done regularly.

As corny as it may sound at the time to the teenager, having the support of other teenagers with diabetes is often a great help. Camps for teenagers with diabetes, often run in the school holidays, are a great way to mix socially with others in the same boat. Often this experience may lead to the adolescent becoming more interested in diabetes self-care as they can share a lot of the same feelings and find out answers to common problems. It is also a good time to have diabetes knowledge updated as a lot is forgotten over the years and often the parents have been the sole carers for their child's diabetes. New advances may have occurred to help improve diabetes care.

Adolescence is a difficult, and often the hardest, time of life for both parents and children alike. Things usually do get better. There are many people with diabetes who have gone from neglecting their diabetes as a teenager to working towards tighter and better control in their maturing years. They often look back, comment on those years with regret and say how much better they feel now, with additional energy, both physically and emotionally.

If the challenges that adolescence presents to the diabetic teenager are understood, it may enable the family to go through this time with less disruption to the diabetes and to the family than otherwise. Most families are pleasantly surprised to see how well the previously rebellious adolescent eventually takes on the responsibility of managing the diabetes and life itself.

Chapter 20

Diabetes and the Elderly

Ten per cent of people over 65 years are aware that they have diabetes. However, even more people have it, but have not been diagnosed. With increasing age, this becomes even more common. This chapter will deal with diabetes care for the elderly, which is arbitrarily defined as those people over 75 years. As our bodies continue to change throughout life, so does the management of diabetes.

In the older age group, people may have the typical symptoms of having diabetes, which are:
- thirst;
- passing lots of urine day and night;
- blurred vision; and
- fatigue.

However, they may also have more unusual symptoms such as:
- loss of appetite;
- incontinence; and
- confusion or drowsiness.

Elderly people may have symptoms from both the short-term or long-term complications of diabetes, which may have been present for a long time without being diagnosed.

Some of the short-term complications which can be dangerous are:
- infections; and
- hyperosmolar coma. This may occur over several days when blood glucose levels become very high and severe dehydration

results. This complication is uncommon. The person becomes progressively more drowsy and may temporarily appear to have had a stroke.

There is usually good recovery with intravenous fluids and insulin treatment. There may be an underlying infection which had precipitated the condition and must also be treated. Excess alcohol and cortisone-type drugs can also precipitate the condition.

The older patient may not have any of the above symptoms typical of diabetes. Instead, one or more of the long-term complications can cause them to seek medical help. Some of these are:

- poor vision (due to diabetic retinopathy, cataracts);
- angina, calf pain on walking, partial or complete stroke, due to hardened and obstructed arteries; and
- numbness, burning in the feet or even ulceration due to peripheral neuropathy.

For more details of chronic complications, *see* chapter 13, 'Avoiding long-term complications'.

AIMS OF TREATMENT

In the same way as in younger people, treatment for diabetes in the older age group is aimed at minimising and controlling the short- and long-term problems associated with diabetes.

CONTROLLING THE SYMPTOMS

By lowering the blood glucose levels, symptoms such as thirst and passing of lots of urine will cease. However, it is important that this does not happen at the cost of making the blood glucose level too low, resulting in hypoglycaemia or a hypo. This is especially important when a person is living alone or is frail.

PREVENTING THE COMPLICATIONS

Problems such as foot ulceration and some forms of eye disease are more common in the older person with diabetes. These problems need special attention and consideration. Regular podiatry and eye review are essential for the older person with diabetes.

HOW TO ACHIEVE THE AIMS OF TREATMENT

1. What has precipitated the diabetes?

A doctor should check that there is no other cause for diabetes developing or worsening in an elderly person. For example, some tablets for blood pressure, bronchitis, arthritis or other inflammatory conditions can raise the blood glucose level. In particular, diuretic or cortisone-like tablets commonly raise the blood glucose level. Infections or other illnesses which decrease activity levels can lead to high blood glucose readings.

2. Education

Ideally, the person with diabetes should take an active role in its management, and so education is important. Sometimes elderly people may have difficulties in acquiring knowledge and learning new skills. These can include difficulty with memory (as can occur with dementia), language barriers or other illnesses. A diabetes educator may help overcome these difficulties by, for example, involving the family or carer in the education, arranging for community nursing care and ensuring adequate medical care of other conditions. Diabetes centres may have an elderly support group which provides social support as well.

3. Nutrition

Diet is important in controlling diabetes regardless of how old or young a person with diabetes is at the time. It is important that an elderly person with diabetes talks with a dietitian, especially if a doctor has asked him or her to make other changes in the diet because of other health problems. The general information available for young people with diabetes is not the right information for the older person with diabetes.

Most elderly people with diabetes still have some insulin production of their own. The problem with the type of diabetes mainly affecting elderly people is that the insulin produced by the body is not able to work efficiently and not enough insulin is released for the body's needs. A diabetic diet in an elderly person does not need to be strictly controlled in terms of timing of meals or the amounts of carbohydrate in each meal (*see* chapter 5, 'Introduction to food'). The diet should be adequate in essential nutrients and suited to the person's circumstances, but some weight loss may be of particular benefit.

4. Exercise

Exercise makes our bodies respond more efficiently to insulin and helps with weight loss. For these reasons, exercise remains an important part of managing diabetes, regardless of a person's age. The exercise intensity needed to achieve the goal of 'metabolic fitness' is still achievable with people who are elderly. Exercise also improves other problems which commonly occur in the elderly, including osteoporosis and high blood pressure. Regular weight-bearing exercise such as walking helps to maintain bone and muscle, and it also improves coordination and helps to prevent falls.

Even walking rather than driving to the shops to get the paper or milk is good exercise. Asking a friend or spouse to come along helps to make the exercise more sociable, safe and fun. Fancy equipment is not needed other than making sure that the shoes are suitable (see below and chapter 14, 'Foot care'). Gentle, enjoyable and regular exercise is better than intense, but rare bouts of exercise.

Other health problems

A check-up with a local doctor is always a good start; sometimes a few tests may be needed. Other health problems may limit the types of exercise. Below are a few suggestions.

Problem	Possible solutions
Osteoarthritis: stiff and painful joints	Warming up and stretching is important at the start of any exercise. Low-impact exercises are better so that musculoskeletal damage is avoided, e.g. walking in a heated pool (check with the local council or the rheumatology department of a local hospital). Stretching exercises help to maintain joint movements (check with a physiotherapist).

Heart or lung conditions: breathlessness on exertion	These need review by a doctor, who may perform a stress test (a person exercises either on a bike or treadmill under the supervision of a doctor, who checks the blood pressure and cardiograph) to see what is a safe distance for the person to walk, swim or cycle.
Difficulty with walking or using a wheelchair e.g. after a stroke	Chair aerobic exercise (videotapes are available).
Peripheral vascular disease or claudication (poor circulation to the legs): pains in the calves on walking	Walking to the onset of the pain is safe and helps to improve the circulation, but this should be discussed with a doctor first. Foot care is very important.
Dementia: confusion, poor memory	These people need to walk with a carer for safety.
Concern about leaving the house	There are exercises for older people available on video which are suitable for doing at home.

5. Tablets which control the blood sugar

These have been discussed in detail in a previous chapter. Illnesses such as liver or kidney disease may influence the type of tablets suitable for a particular person to take. In an elderly person, doses are started in small amounts and increased very slowly. Since a low blood glucose level can occur if too much of a blood glucose lowering tablet is taken, it is always important that the correct dose of tablet be used. Since elderly people are frequently taking many different tablets, a dosette box can be very useful to help people remember when to take the tablets. If a new tablet is started, it is important that the doctor is aware of the current treatment for the diabetes. During bouts of illness, the doctor should advise the elderly person on how to deal with these medications (*see* chapter 12, 'The highs of diabetes', for sick day advice).

6. Insulin

The form of diabetes which is always treated with insulin occurs in children and young adults (insulin dependent diabetes — IDDM). However, a small number of people older than 70 years of age are also treated with insulin. Many older people start insulin treatment when tablets are no longer enough to keep the blood glucose level in the right range. This is not a sign of failure in the person or that the diabetes is becoming more dangerous, but rather that the pancreas is not making enough insulin for the body's needs. Again, a doctor and diabetes educator would look at what type of insulin is best for that particular person's needs. Elderly people with diabetes who start insulin treatment often need large amounts of insulin to control the blood glucose, especially compared to the smaller doses that a young person with diabetes might need. The correct dose is the dose that makes the blood glucose normal — no matter how small or large.

Other health problems may affect an elderly person's ability to cope with insulin, but there are ways of tackling all these problems so that independence can be maintained.

Problem	Possible solutions
Poor eyesight: difficulty with blood testing or insulin injection	Good lighting Magnifying glass Insulin pens that click to make it easy to count
Tremor or stroke (shakes)	Single-hand drawing-up devices or insulin pens
Arthritis	Insulin pens
Dementia/memory problems	Family member or community sister can draw up insulin

If drawing up and injecting insulin is a particular problem, it is sometimes wise for the elderly to use a longer-acting insulin so that a 'once a day' injection is enough to keep the blood glucose under reasonable control.

7. Other problems for older people

Where there are problems there are always solutions.

Problem	Possible solutions
Poor mobility: limited ability to attend for medical care or to do shopping	Community bus Taxi subsidy Home deliveries Family or friends to help out
Poor dentures — less food choice	Advice from dentist or dental hospital
Financial limitations	Social worker for advice about possible assistance
Lack of cooking knowledge	Adult education classes St Vincent's Diabetes Cookbook has simple, tasty recipes which are easy to follow
Difficulty cooking due to arthritis or poor vision	Meals On Wheels can deliver special diets (e.g. diabetic) if requested

PREVENTING COMPLICATIONS

Knowing a person has diabetes makes it easier to prevent complications such as hyperosmolar coma as described earlier in this chapter. Carrying a diabetes identification card is useful to ensure that, if any emergency occurs, medical personnel are aware of the presence of diabetes.

Blood glucose tests by the elderly person at home or by a family member, local doctor or community nurse provide a warning system if problems are occurring with diabetes. A higher blood glucose reading may indicate that there is a hidden infection or another illness has become unstable, such as heart failure or angina. It is important, therefore, that a sudden rise in blood glucose levels in an elderly person be reviewed by medical personnel.

In an elderly person with diabetes, a low blood glucose level can be more dangerous than an occasional high blood glucose reading. For this reason, a higher blood glucose level may be acceptable in some people because of the emphasis placed on avoiding the problem of hypoglycaemia. For someone treated with diet alone, there is no risk of a low blood glucose. Also, people treated with metformin tablets on their own are unlikely to get serious hypoglycaemia. Since the long-term problems of diabetes due to high blood glucose levels may not develop for several years, there is less need for 'tight' control in someone who is elderly, (i.e. less need to keep the blood glucose in the normal range). Blood glucose levels should be kept as close to normal as possible, however, in order to keep the elderly person symptom-free and safe from infection or dehydration.

Looking after diabetes well in the longer term can help prevent future problems. Diabetic complications are discussed in chapter 13, 'Avoiding long-term complications'. Atherosclerosis is one such disease which affects the heart (with the risk of angina and heart attacks), the legs (with the risk of peripheral vascular disease) and the blood vessels to the brain (with the risk of stroke). These potential problems are tackled by having reasonable control of diabetes, but also by controlling potential other risk factors for artery disease.

Problem	Possible solutions
Risk factor for atherosclerosis	Action needed in an elderly person with diabetes
Smoking	You are never too old to stop (or too foolish to continue) and it is never too late to get the benefit from stopping.
Hypertension (high blood pressure)	Studies have shown that even 'very elderly' people benefit from treatment of high blood pressure — it still lowers the risk of stroke and heart disease.
Cholesterol and triglyceride levels	These are less important as a risk factor as we get older, so tablets are not always needed; fat in the diet still needs to be controlled.

Family history of heart disease	People whose parents had heart disease have a greater risk themselves and should be more active in preventing it.

Aside from atherosclerosis, other potential problems related to diabetes need care. Eye care is as important in older people as in young people, especially since poor vision can limit independence. Eye problems such as glaucoma and cataracts are the most common in elderly people and may need treatment. Regular checks with an eye specialist (yearly to second-yearly on average, but more often if it is required) will achieve this goal.

Since older age groups are more likely to have other health problems, it is always important for an elderly person to let those helping to look after their health know about their diabetes, e.g. when being admitted to hospital or seeing another doctor or a new community nurse.

The fact that someone has reached older age is a good sign that they have the skills to deal with diabetes. With appropriate care, a healthy, active life can be enjoyed into old age despite diabetes.

References
The Diabetes Centre, St Vincent's Hospital, Sydney, *Diabetes and ageing: A guide to management and education,* 1992.

Chapter 21

Eating Away From Home

This chapter outlines how to enjoy takeaway food and dining out, and still make healthy food choices, after developing diabetes.

Eating out is one of the great joys of life. It is estimated that more than 30% of the family food budget is spent on foods consumed away from home. There is no reason a person cannot continue to frequent a favourite restaurant, enjoy takeaway food or accept dinner invitations after having been diagnosed with diabetes.

The first question to ask is how often do you eat away from home? If it is only once a year — well, let your hair down and enjoy everything! However, is you are eating away from home two to three times a week, think much more carefully about what types of foods to choose from the menu.

RESTAURANTS

Always start by reading the menu carefully and asking the waiter or waitress if you are unable to understand anything. Also ask the waiter to explain what sauces or dressings come with the dish and what to expect by way of accompaniments, e.g., vegetables, salad, bread. By getting all this information before choosing the food, it is possible to make the most appropriate choice.

It is difficult to keep to the normal routine of a low-fat diet with restaurant meals. The chef has gone to a lot of trouble to make the dish taste and look as good as possible — and more often than not this means lots of fat. Do the best possible in a difficult situation. If regular eating our is a problem, discuss this with a dietitian for individual advice.

HOW MANY COURSES?

This is a good questions to ask. The first thing many of my clients say to me is, 'Well, only two because you can't have dessert when you've got diabetes.' I would agree with the two courses, but not the reason. Read the menu carefully — perhaps there is a dessert which contains less fat than all the entrées do. From reading the chapter on food, it is seen that sugar is not such a 'baddy' as previously thought. Extra sugar in the form of dessert will not have such bad long-term consequences as having lots of fat. Sugar, by weight, has less kilojoules than fat, so for those watching their weight this is an important consideration.

Good examples of low-fat food choices can be found at the end of this chapter.

> Julie loved to eat out at least twice a week. Tonight she was at a new restaurant with her friends from work, so she wasn't very familiar with the food. Everyone gave her some good-natured teasing when she kept asking the waiter a lot of questions, but Julie just laughed them off — they weren't the ones who were going to have an awful hypo at 2 a.m. if they didn't eat enough carbohydrate! The entrée list was awful — deep-fried calamari, cream of broccoli soup, antipasto plate and pâté. She gave the entrée a miss. The mains offered a good selection and the meal came with crusty bread and a salad. The desserts looked promising; the choices included rockmelon sorbet and strawberries in Grand Marnier — both better choices than those entrées. Tonight, rockmelon sorbet was the choice and she decided not to take up the offer of an accompanying dollop of cream.

HOW FUSSY CAN I BE?

So, you want the avocado seafood *without* the thousand island dressing and you want the side salad *without* the olive oil and you want the blueberries *without* cream. Is the chef going to be upset? Well, most restaurants will be quite happy to accommodate this request. If not, go to a different restaurant to find one which will.

WHAT ABOUT ALCOHOL?

A few facts about alcohol:
1. One standard drink, i.e. 1 middy beer, 1 nip of spirits, 1 small glass of wine, all contain approximately the same kilojoules, i.e. equal to 270 kJ. If you are watching your weight, try to keep to one or two drinks and be popular by volunteering to drive everyone home.
2. Low-alcohol beers contain a little more residual sugar, but are somewhat lower in energy.
3. Most alcoholic beverages contain virtually no residual sugar. The exception is alcoholic cider and some speciality brands of beer.
4. Alcohol can cause hypoglycaemia, especially in people taking insulin so it is best to have alcohol with a meal. Alcohol is a common contributing cause of overnight hypos after a night out. It may be necessary to decrease the amount of insulin and/or eat extra carbohydrate to prevent this from occurring. If you have more questions about this, contact the local diabetes educator and/or dietitian for individual advice.

TAKEAWAYS

Takeaway food outlets fall into two broad categories. First, there are the big chains, e.g. McDonald's, KFC, Pizza Hut etc. Secondly, there are the myriad of small businesses selling sandwiches, hamburgers, fish and chips, Thai, Indian food, etc.

With the first group, the advice is to be very careful. These outlets sell very high fat foods. Also, the type of fat they use is not polyunsaturated or monounsaturated, and consequently is the worst type of fat to consume. Just consider these few facts:

Type of takeaway food	g fat
Big Mac, 1 burger	27.0
McDonald's Chicken Nugget, 1 serve	20.5
McDonald's Fries, 1 medium serve	20.0
Pizza Hut Pizza, ½ deep pan Supreme	24.5
McDonald's milkshake, 1 large	15.0
KFC Chicken Fillet Burger	22.5
Chiko Roll, 1	17.5

(Reference: Rosemary Stanton's *Fat and Fibre Counter*, Wilkinson Books, 1993.)

With the small outlets, let the skills which have been learnt from restaurant meals go to work. For example:
- Ask the fish shop to grill rather than deep fry the fish.
- Choose boiled rice instead of fried rice.
- Choose baked naan bread rather than deep-fried pappadams.
- Ask for a plain hamburger rather than one with the lot.
- Get the sandwich hand to go easy on the margarine and mayonnaise, or ask for no spread.
- Find a Thai restaurant that only uses polyunsaturated vegetable oil for cooking.

Many places now also sell prepared salads, crusty rolls and ready-made fruit desserts: all great, healthy foods with all the convenience of takeaway.

DINNER PARTIES AND OTHER CELEBRATIONS

These can be difficult times for those trying to do the right thing. Again, put the celebration into perspective to decide how vigilant you need to be. If it is the third party in a week, be a bit more careful than if it is the first wedding you have been to in years.
- Obviously, there is little that can be done about the type of food served, so perhaps be wary about the quantities eaten. If it is a buffet, make the best choices possible and fill up on plenty of rice- or pasta-based dishes and bread. This way you will feel full and may find it easier to have only a small plate of chocolate mousse for dessert.
- If going to dinner at a friend's house is a problem, practise saying no to seconds, but still giving due praise to the meal, e.g. 'That was so delicious, to have anymore would spoil what I have already enjoyed.'
- If there is a choice, ask for smaller serves, then, if feeling obliged to have seconds, you haven't had too much to begin with. Beware of pre-dinner 'nibbles' — these are often high in fat. Try to save up until dinner. Perhaps offer to bring a dessert for everyone. Many of the new low-fat cookbooks available contain recipes for simple but delicious low-fat desserts which would complement even the most elaborate meals. It doesn't have to be fruit salad every time.

Remember, many Australians are trying to eat a healthy diet whether they have diabetes or not. Most people are happy to experiment with new and exciting low-fat recipes at all your dinner parties. Maybe people will be converted when shown that low-fat eating does not have to be boring.

GETTING THE TIMING OF TABLETS/INSULIN RIGHT WHEN GOING OUT

This can often be a problem when the usual evening meal time is usually 6 p.m. and it is known that no one eats at the Jones's until at least 9 p.m. Some people, especially those on tablets, do not worry about the time difference and find that their blood glucose levels are just fine. Others find it a big problem.

Some suggestions

1. Have the tablets/insulin at the normal time and then have the usual supper snack to eat before going out. Then it is safe to eat the main meal many hours later knowing that a hypo is unlikely to happen. To fill up before the party may also help decrease overconsumption later.
2. Some people on insulin prefer to wait until they know they are going to eat before having the injection. If this is preferred, that is fine. A quick exit just when dinner goes on the table to give your injection will be quite unnoticeable. Conversely, many people are comfortable injecting at the table. In restaurants, it can be more tricky as some people feel uncomfortable about injecting themselves in the toilets. You may prefer suggestion 1. If this is regularly a problem, talk to a diabetes educator about having an insulin pen instead of syringes, which can be a more unobtrusive way to deliver the insulin.
3. If adjusting insulin doses, do not forget to find out what food is to be eaten beforehand so as to know exactly what adjustments need to be made.
4. If it is going to be a long or late night, people on a pre-bed insulin dose may wish to take this with them so that the injection time stays similar to normal. Remember, if up all night dancing, less insulin will be needed and perhaps more food.

Speak to a diabetes educator for individual advice if problems persist.

WHAT TO DRINK?

Here are some ideas on how to stick to only a few alcoholic drinks for the evening.

1. Use lots of low-joule mixers and ice in drinks to make them go further.
2. Try ½ nips, rather than full nips of spirits.
3. Sparkling mineral water, soda water or low-joule tonic go well with white wine to make a 'spritzer'. It has half the energy of a full glass, but you can feel like you have been keeping up with everyone else.
4. Try a non-alcoholic drink in between each alcoholic drink.
5. Drink low-alcohol beer.
6. Choose middies of beer rather than schooners.
7. If going to someone else's house, always take some low-joule drinks in case they don't serve anything suitable.
8. Beware of drinking too much fruit juice! Each 250 mL glass of juice contains 380 kJ; this can certainly add up over an evening. However, if taking insulin and concerned about going hypo while dancing and/or drinking alcohol, fruit juice may be an easy way to get more carbohydrate.
9. Vegetable juices are often a good alternative to fruit juice. Tomato juice with a dash of Worcestershire or Tabasco sauce is a very refreshing and low-energy drink!

EATING AWAY FROM HOME – A QUICK GUIDE TO FOOD CHOICES

Aussie style

Wise choices	*Poor choices*
BBQ chicken (skin removed)	Deep-fried chicken
Grilled fish/seafood	Deep-fried fish/seafood
Plain hamburger with salad	Hamburger with the lot
Filled rolls and sandwiches	Chiko rolls, spring rolls, battered sausages
Doner kebab/felafel	Meat pie, sausage roll
Steak sandwich	
Jacket potato	Chips, potato scallops

Asian

Wise choices
- Steamed dim sim
- Wonton bun
- Soups
- San choy bow
- Steamed/braised/BBQ/ Stir-fried dishes

- Seafood, chicken, lean meat, vegetables

- Steamed rice/noodles

Poor choices
- Deep-fried spring rolls
- Puffs, wonton, prawn toast

- Deep-fried/battered dishes with sweet sauce

- Lemon chicken, sweet and sour pork
- Duck in plum sauce
- Honey prawns
- Fried rice/noodles
- Dishes with coconut milk/coconut cream

Mediterranean style

Wise choices
- Minestrone
- Grilled/fresh seafood/fish
- Stuffed vegetables
- Veal — wine, lemon, mushroom, tomato sauces
- Bean dishes
- Pasta — Neapolitan, marinara, spinach

Poor choices
- Cream soups
- Deep-fried seafood/fish
- Garlic bread

- Veal in cream sauce

- Carbonara and and ricotta, Bolognese, pesto other cream sauces

Mexican

Wise choices
- Bean dip
- Guacamole
- Mixed vegetable platters and salad
- Soft flour tortilla or taco
- Grilled/BBQ — seafood, chicken, meat
- Legume dishes

Poor choices
- Corn chips
- Sour cream
- Deep-fried tortilla

- Deep-fried seafood, chicken, meat

Lebanese

Wise choices
Yoghurt and bean dip
with Lebanese bread
Lebanese bread
Stuffed vegetables
Salads — tabouleh, etc.
Felafel/kibbi/hofta
Shish/doner kebab

Poor choices
Creamy dips

Deep-fried vegetables

Chapter 22

Who Should Be Told?

Some people like to keep things to themselves, whereas others are more open and do not mind the whole world knowing the state of their health. However, after diagnosis of diabetes there are authorities who **should** be notified, and some whom it would be advisable to inform. This chapter discusses why these people should be notified and what the benefits will be.

WHO SHOULD BE TOLD?

1. Road Traffic Authorities

People who hold any type of driver's licence (be it for private use or for carrying passengers, e.g. for buses) must notify their licensing authority.

It is possible for diabetes to have an impact on a person's health by increasing the risk of accidents. For example, if a driver has an episode of hypoglycaemia (low blood glucose) while driving, there is a serious risk of an accident occurring. Judgment will be impaired and the person can lose consciousness if the hypoglycaemia is not picked up and treated immediately. When the blood glucose level is high (hyperglycaemia), it can cause drowsiness, making it easy for the driver to fall asleep at the wheel. Also, long-term complications can affect the eyes (diabetic retinopathy). This can reduce the field of vision, so that driving becomes hazardous.

Medical reviews required for people with diabetes seeking their driving licence do vary from State to State and to clarify the situation for our readers, we have outlined below the current NSW regulations governed by the *Roads and Traffic Authority*.

Holders of **Class 1A and R licences** will be required to have a medical review every two years instead of every year if they are insulin dependent. If their diabetes is controlled by tablets, the period between medical reviews will be extended to five years instead of the present two years.

Holders of **Class 1B, 3A, 3B, 4A, 4B, 5A, 5B or 5C licences** will have a medical review every year instead of every two years if they use tablets to control their diabetes. If they are insulin dependent, they will continue to be reviewed annually.

2. Health insurance companies

A person with diabetes cannot be denied private health insurance just on the basis of having diabetes. It is likely, however, that a 1-year waiting period will be imposed before the insurance becomes effective (i.e. diabetes is a pre-existing ailment).

If diabetes is diagnosed shortly after joining a health fund, but the person had symptoms prior to joining, then the fund would still consider the diabetes a pre-existing ailment and may impose the 1-year waiting period.

3. Life insurance companies

It is up to each individual life insurance company whether or not to accept someone who has diabetes. It is not a requirement of law to accept everyone who applies. Again, it is important to shop around to get the best possible deal. It is likely that a higher premium will be charged for people with diabetes. Seeking insurance early, maintaining good diabetes control and following a healthy lifestyle may improve the chances of finding satisfactory insurance.

4. Health professionals

It is not unusual to receive medical attention from a number of sources such as doctors, nurses, dietitians, dentists, podiatrists etc. It is important that each health professional knows that you have diabetes, so appropriate care can be given.

If new medication is prescribed, a test ordered or surgery planned, its effects on diabetes should be considered.

WHOM IS IT ADVISABLE TO TELL?

1. At home

The people we live with are our main source of support. Knowledge of what diabetes is, and how it is treated, will allow them to understand better the implications of having diabetes. It also means they can act appropriately in an emergency, such as hypoglycaemia. Doctors, diabetes educators and dietitians are generally happy for people with diabetes to bring a friend or relative to appointments or education sessions.

2. At work

Working environments differ greatly. At work, there is often quite a mixed group of people, some of whom one may trust, others not as much. It is advisable to tell one's employer about the diagnosis of diabetes, for a number of reasons. People with diabetes should eat at fairly regular times. If the workload means that meal times could be delayed, permission (if permission is needed) to have a snack whilst on the job should be sought. Shift workers should seek advice about how to manage their insulin and meals when their hours keep changing. Advice can be obtained from doctors, dietitians and diabetes educators.

Sometimes high blood glucose levels can cause more frequent visits to the toilet to pass urine. Some employers may want to know why their employee keeps disappearing. If employers and co-workers have knowledge of diabetes and hypoglycaemia, they may be able to help in the case of a hypoglycaemic episode. Some employers may be reassured if they see that a person with diabetes is regularly testing the blood glucose levels and generally looking after him/herself.

People who operate heavy or potentially dangerous equipment or work on scaffolding or work with chemicals should consider any risk to themselves and others if they experience hypoglycaemia.

It is a good idea to discuss where and how often insulin injections and blood glucose tests will be done. If the working environment is very hot, a cool place should be organised to keep insulin, e.g. the first aid room or a locker.

In many factories, there are regulations about wearing of safety shoes in some areas. It is very important that those safety shoes have a perfect fit. Poorly fitting shoes can cause serious injuries to the feet (*see* chapter 14, 'Foot care'). If the safety shoes offered by the factory do not fit well, alternative shoes should be found. If that is not possible, the employee may need to be transferred to an area where safety shoes are not worn.

It is not suggested that everyone at work must be told about the diagnosis of diabetes. However, it is advisable to tell some key people, e.g. employer, the first aid officer (if there is one) and a trusted friend or two.

3. Friends or neighbours

People who live alone may want to inform their neighbours about diabetes. Telling a good friend about the condition and the appropriate treatment for hypoglycaemia is a good idea.

4. Sporting groups/clubs

Life is for living. These days, people with diabetes are involved in just about everything. If, however, you are participating in a sport which could have an element of risk, stop and think about whether anyone should be told about the diabetes. For example, those who are avid fishermen and spend long hours in a boat or fishing off rocks may consider whether to do this alone. What will happen if hypoglycaemia occurs? This question would apply to a number of other sports such as surfing or skiing. Participation in sports should still be enjoyed after diagnosis of diabetes, but prior consideration should be taken to do so as safely as possible.

There are some sports in which people rely on each other for safety. In that case, the people should be aware of what to look for and how to deal with emergencies in diabetes. Sugar should be carried at all times and regular eating times should be kept. Often extra carbohydrate should be eaten before exercise and testing of blood glucose levels.

Identification

It is essential to carry some form of identification stating the type of diabetes and the current treatment. There are bracelets, necklaces and cards for placing in a wallet or purse available from pharmacies, diabetes centres and Diabetes Australia.

Postscript

There are some professions denied to people with diabetes, e.g. airline pilot and scuba diving instructor. If looking to start in a new career, it is wise to find out if diabetes will be a problem. Diabetes Australia can be of assistance when negotiating with prospective employers or professional bodies.

Chapter 23

Travel and Diabetes

This chapter describes the pitfalls of travel for the person with diabetes – and how to avoid or deal with them. Travelling is one of the most exciting, fun-filled and delightful experiences that anyone can have. However, some people with diabetes deny themselves this experience. Quite often the reasons given are that it is too much trouble or there is a fear of the problems that may occur, e.g. hypoglycaemia in an unknown environment.

It does not matter whether diabetes is controlled by diet, tablets or insulin, there is no reason to miss travel to any location in the world. The main thing needed is some extra planning and organisation to make sure a holiday for a person with diabetes goes ahead smoothly.

One of the first things that should be arranged is a review with the doctor caring for diabetes, and/or your diabetes educator. The role of these people is to provide information so that planning and preparation for some of the feared perils that may be faced on a journey can be made. Part of the planning involves being aware of the challenges that may lie ahead:
- delayed flights;
- lost luggage;
- jet lag;
- traveller's diarrhoea;
- unfamiliar foods;
- change in activity;
- changes in temperatures;
- lengthy sightseeing tours; and
- running out of insulin.

There are many types of transport around the world, but for each form there may be a need to take along different things in order to be organised for the days ahead of you. It may take a little longer to do, but it will make the trip much easier, especially if things do not go smoothly.

The following are questions that people often ask when contemplating travel. Many of the questions asked are not thought of until the holiday is well under way, out of the reach of the diabetes team. So, whether the diabetes is controlled by diet, tablets or insulin, answering these questions before the trip may help the travel go smoothly.

WHAT TO DO IN PREPARATION FOR TRAVELLING?

At least one month before travelling, it is important to see the doctor and check that diabetes control and general health are satisfactory. If there are changes to be made to the treatment, there is still time before travelling. Early planning reduces the worry about medical problems at the last moment.

ARE MEDICAL LETTERS OF INTRODUCTION NECESSARY?

It is a good idea to have a letter from the doctor describing recent medical problems and current treatment. Then, if medical treatment is sought while travelling, current problems and care are fully explained in the accompanying letter.

If taking insulin, a letter is necessary stating that there is a need to carry insulin, syringes and a glucose meter. This will help at customs counters in airports. This letter is specifically for customs when leaving or entering different countries. It is not required when travelling within Australia.

If staying in any particular country for an extended period of time, it may be necessary to ask the doctor for a contact name and address of a diabetes specialist overseas. If the local doctor is unable to provide a contact person, make contact with the Australian consulate in that particular country if problems do occur. The consulate should be able to provide the name of an English-speaking doctor who will be able to help.

WHEN SHOULD VACCINATIONS BE GIVEN, IF NEEDED?

Again, ask the local doctor, but it is important to have the vaccinations done early (at least 1 month prior to departure). This will allow time for the protecting antibodies to be made in the body, and allow time to recover if the control of diabetes is affected for a short period.

SHOULD AN IDENTITY BRACELET OR CHAIN BE WORN?

Yes, especially if on medication. These are a very valuable item to have, and are available from Diabetes Australia. Identification chains and bracelets can help in case of an emergency and are a good form of identification in Australia as well.

WHAT ABOUT TRAVEL INSURANCE?

Obtaining insurance today is a lot easier for people with diabetes than it has been previously. Having travel insurance is an essential part of the preparation for travelling, especially when going overseas. Diabetes Australia is able to provide the names of companies which insure for diabetes related-illnesses, as well as other chronic medical problems.

If the person with diabetes is already a member of a health fund, it is worthwhile inquiring about travel insurance. Some health funds provide a discount to members already insured with them. However, they may charge an extra amount in the case of diabetes. Always be aware of any special conditions the company may have in regards to taking out a policy. For example, any treatment for a pre-existing condition by a doctor 60 days prior to travel can allow the company to charge an extra fee.

It is important to remember that the policy should be read thoroughly before signing and accepting the conditions. Be aware of any further costs that may be incurred if the policy agreement is not adhered to, or broken. It is a good idea to look at the various policies available; do not just take out the first policy that is offered.

WHAT ABOUT INSULIN/TABLETS AND OTHER MEDICATIONS?

If travelling overseas, it is a good idea to obtain a script for twice the amount of insulin and/or tablets that would be normally used during the time of the holiday. A script for glucagon, and all other medications that the doctor thinks necessary, should also be filled at the chemist before departure; these may include antidiarrhoeals and antibiotics. It is necessary to be prepared for most eventualities.

WHAT PRECAUTIONS ARE NEEDED WHEN TRAVELLING BY CAR, BUS OR TRAIN?

- Stop for short breaks and take time out for a short walk. As the campaign from the NSW Road and Traffic Authority (RTA) states, 'Stop, revive, survive.'
- Do not drink alcohol.
- Have snacks and meals on time.
- Carry extra food and drink in the car, or in hand luggage on a train or bus, in case of delays on the road or a missed meal.
- If taking insulin and/or tablets, treat the symptoms of hypoglycaemia straight away. The car should be stopped. If the driver develops a hypo, he or she should get out from behind the wheel so there is no temptation to start driving the car before being fully recovered from the episode.
- Carry or wear identification at all times.
- It is also a good idea to carry quick-acting carbohydrates such as soft drinks (not low-calorie), glucose tablets or sugar cubes. Also, carry longer acting carbohydrate such as sandwiches, Morning Coffee biscuits or some fruit to follow up the initial quick-acting carbohydrate in case of a hypoglycaemic episode.

SHOULD THE AIRLINE OR TRAVEL COMPANY BE NOTIFIED THAT A PERSON HAS DIABETES?

When travelling by plane, people with diabetes usually receive their meals first. Sometimes, they are also given a greater choice regarding seat positions, i.e. whether it is an aisle seat or near to the toilets.

IS IT NECESSARY TO ORDER SPECIAL MEALS ON THE PLANE?

Again, this is not absolutely necessary. A selection of suitable meals is usually possible from the meals already available to the other passengers.

HOW SHOULD INSULIN BE CARRIED ON THE PLANE?

It is always handy to keep a double supply of insulin and monitoring equipment. One set in the hand luggage, and the other in ordinary luggage. If travelling with a friend, share some of the supplies and equipment. Some people have had the unfortunate problem of landing at their destination, e.g. Paris, and finding out that their luggage and diabetes treatment arrived in New York.

Insulin remains stable in a refrigerator for approximately 2 years, depending on the use-by-date on each of the vials. When insulin is taken out of the refrigerator and is left at 20°C–25°C it remains stable for 1 month before it needs to be disposed of. Insulin should not become frozen or exposed to warm temperatures, as it will lose much of its action. Some people prefer to carry the insulin in an insulated pack or in a vacuum flask containing cold water.

HOW IS INSULIN INJECTED ON THE PLANE?

There is a lowered air pressure on the plane, so it is necessary to put only half the amount of air into the vial. That is, if the regular insulin dose required is 30 units, then put in 15 units of air into the vial before drawing up the intended insulin.

HOW ARE INSULIN/TABLETS ADJUSTED FOR TIME ZONE CHANGES?

First, discuss this with the doctor and/or diabetes educator. There are different ways of adjusting insulin when travelling through time zones. To help with this, it is advisable to monitor blood glucose levels every 6 hours in all situations. Two common approaches that the doctor and educator may suggest are:
1. Keeping to 'home time' while on the plane. On arriving at the destination, switch over to the local time, reducing the insulin

dose if there is an overlap. For example, when arriving in London at 8 a.m. (5 p.m. Australian Eastern standard time), test the blood glucose level and then give a dose of insulin somewhat less than the usual morning dose. The insulin dose may need to be modified in relation to the blood glucose level at the time of the dose.
2. Take short-acting insulin every 6 hours, i.e. before each meal offered on the plane, monitoring the blood glucose level prior to each of these meals to enable an appropriate dose to be determined; a guideline to the dose is to take approximately one-quarter of the usual total daily insulin dose before each meal (at 5–8 hourly intervals) with a slight increase or decrease to the blood glucose level. On arriving at the destination, the usual regimen can be recommenced. Again, remember the first dose of usual insulin may need to be adjusted for the current blood glucose level.

HOW SOON BEFORE A MEAL SHOULD INSULIN BE INJECTED?

The best idea is not to inject the insulin until the meal tray arrives at the seat, sometimes food can be delayed because of unforeseen circumstances, e.g. air turbulence. It is important to keep this in mind so that problems do not occur such as a hypoglycaemic episode because the insulin has been injected, but the food did not arrive as expected. Similarly, at restaurants, insulin should only be injected when the meal has arrived.

WHAT IF AIRSICKNESS OCCURS ON THE PLANE?

One of the easiest ways to deal with this is to keep a can of soft drink, and sip it slowly, especially if solid foods cannot be kept down. Follow the 'sick day' guidelines previously discussed with the diabetes educator, dietitian and/or doctor (*see* chapter 12, 'The highs of diabetes').

WHAT TO DO IF A HYPO OCCURS?

It is important to keep adequate carbohydrate in the hand luggage. That way, even if there is a delay in the lounge at the airport, there is sufficient carbohydrate available to replace a meal.

If travelling with a friend, it is a good idea to educate him or her about hypos, and to carry glucagon, as well as knowing how to give it, if necessary. It is a safe way of raising the blood glucose level in someone who is uncooperative or unconscious. This will enable the person to recover enough to take some carbohydrate orally.

HOW CAN SWELLING IN THE LEGS BE PREVENTED OR EASED WHILST ON THE PLANE?

The most helpful thing to do is to keep the feet elevated from the floor, and try to walk as often as possible to help with circulation. There are several things that can be done to aid this:
- Use a push-cush, which is an air cushion to help elevate and exercise the feet (available from chemists and Diabetes Australia).
- Do foot exercises while sitting down.
- Do not forget to wear comfortable shoes, preferably lace-up style, to allow for some swelling of the feet.

IMPORTANT POINTS TO REMEMBER ONCE ARRIVING AT EACH DESTINATION

Not all countries throughout the world have the same strength of insulin as in Australia. In Australia, the strength of insulin is 100 units per mL. Some countries use a combination of 40 units per mL, as well as 100 units per mL. If there is a need to obtain insulin while travelling, check the strength of the insulin before purchasing. One of the easiest ways to deal with this, if the holiday involves only travelling to three or four places, is to contact the company who manufactures the insulin that is being used. Then, find out what strength of insulin is sold in those particular countries, and where the insulin can be purchased. If uncertain about doing any of this, contact the local diabetes centre, who will be able to help.

WHAT IF THE INSULIN TAKEN OVERSEAS RUNS OUT AND MORE NEEDS TO BE PURCHASED?

If the 40 units per mL from certain countries is the only available insulin, it is essential to use the U-40 syringes from that country with this insulin so that the markings on the syringe correspond to the units of insulin that are to be given.

Once again, the best idea is to tell the diabetes educator before travel begins which countries are to be visited. Then, find out which company makes your particular insulin, and if the company has a reciprocal company in the country to be visited. By doing this, if insulin is to be purchased, all the preparations will have been done so that you know the availability of the insulin in the particular countries and from where to obtain it.

Diabetes Australia can also supply further information and resources (particularly contact addresses for similar diabetes associations, e.g. in the UK and the USA). The consulates for the different countries can also supply information about hospitals, insulin supplies and other specific needs.

Be warned: Even if you make arrangements to purchase insulin or other pharmaceutical supplies overseas, they are likely to be very much more expensive than in Australia – so try to take sufficient surplus to last through the trip.

WHAT IF A GASTRIC UPSET DEVELOPS?

It is vital that, if food cannot be eaten, insulin is not omitted. Use the sick day management that would be followed at home, which has been discussed with your doctor, diabetes educator and/or dietitian. Flat ordinary soft drink can be used as a form of carbohydrate and adequate fluid intake must be maintained so that dehydration does not occur. Monitor blood glucose levels frequently and check urine for ketones (this is for people who are insulin controlled), (*see* chapter 4, 'Assessment of diabetes control').

Contact a doctor if vomiting or nausea persists, if oral fluids cannot be taken or if high blood glucose levels or ketones in the urine develop.

Some general principles to help avoid a stomach upset are as follows:
- Drink only bottled water (or water that has been boiled).
- Avoid ice.
- Avoid raw vegetables and fruit, unless they are peeled by you at the time of eating.

WHAT COULD MAKE DIABETES CONTROL UNSTABLE WHEN TRAVELLING?

Let's face it, when travelling there are a lot of different things happening which can affect the body, including jet lag, unfamiliar meals, travel sickness and excitement. The only way to keep a check on the blood glucose level is to test frequently and to make temporary adjustments in insulin doses.

Becoming a tourist often mean an increase in exercise, e.g. walking while sightseeing, extra sports, walking to transport. This extra exercise may result in hypoglycaemia if the diabetes is controlled with insulin and/or tablets. A different diet may lead to a different amount of carbohydrate. A dietitian/educator can advise about carbohydrate choices in other countries.

If on a bus or train, carry adequate carbohydrate in case of delays, causing missed or late meals.

HOW CAN FOOT TROUBLE BE AVOIDED WHEN TRAVELLING?

Take extra care of feet by wearing 'broken-in' comfortable shoes. This is not the time to start wearing a brand new pair of shoes. Never go barefoot, particularly on hot sand or on pebbles at the beach. Check the feet every day for blisters, cuts or abrasions. If these happen, use iodine or an antiseptic solution, and a gauze dressing and paper nonstick tape. Carry these simple treatments with you.

If any foot problems are being experienced before travelling, it is a good idea to see the podiatrist prior to commencing the holiday. The podiatrist will also be able to provide, or show how to use, protective foam rubber or shoe inserts to protect pressure-vulnerable areas.

Now go ahead and enjoy yourself.

Easy-to-put-together travel kit

For both insulin dependent diabetes mellitus (IDDM) and non-insulin dependent diabetes mellitus (NIDDM)
- Iodine solution (antiseptic for cuts, blisters) and a simple nonstick dressing.
- Test strips, lancets, Keto-diastix (IDDM only).
- Blood glucose meter.

- Medications for diabetes and/or other conditions.
- Thermometer and paracetamol.
- Carbohydrate for hypoglycaemia treatment: soft drink, jelly beans, dried fruits, plain biscuits.

In addition for insulin treated people:
- Syringes – double the amount that is needed.
- If using a pen, take a second one, plus some syringes in case the devices break or are lost.
- Insulin – double the amount needed. Share this with a friend and carry some in hand luggage.
- Syringe disposal unit, e.g. empty soft drink screw top bottle.
- Glucagon for injection.

Chapter 24

Research in Diabetes Mellitus

In the 75 years since insulin was discovered, enormous strides have been made in the treatment of diabetes mellitus, but the goals of prevention and cure remain elusive. Whilst this is being sought, research continues to improve diabetes management so as to ensure the prevention of complications of diabetes mellitus.

BLOOD GLUCOSE MONITORING, INSULIN DELIVERY AND FORMULATIONS

A normal pancreas is constantly sampling the blood glucose level and receiving readings to allow it to anticipate meal-related blood glucose rises, so that appropriate adjustment to insulin secretion can be made. It is impossible with current home blood glucose monitoring to do this as often as the pancreas does. Sampling of the interstitium (space between various cells of the body) glucose levels may provide an improvement by allowing more frequent glucose sampling. The information on glucose levels obtained from such a sampling device could be used in a feedback loop using a computer system to determine appropriate adjustments to insulin secretion rate from an insulin delivery system.

Insulin produced by the pancreas is released into portal circulation, i.e. into the blood directly travelling to the liver. Subcutaneous administration, either via a pump or via injections, leads to high insulin levels systemically (throughout the body), not just in the portal system, which is not ideal. Delivery systems which release insulin into the portal circulation, e.g. via a peritoneal catheter (delivery tubing feeding into abdominal cavity), may provide a more physiological way of insulin administration. Problems with infection, catheter blockage and computer malfunction still need to be resolved before such means of insulin release become available.

The future is likely to bring different types of insulin for injection, e.g. other ways of extending the action of insulin than the current crystallisation methods. This will lead to smoother and more predictable insulin release. The coupling of such preparations to the newer quicker onset insulins will lead to better control.

Since insulin is a protein, it cannot be taken by mouth since it would be destroyed by the digestive enzymes of the intestine. Research continues into agents which are able to be taken orally and be absorbed, and subsequently act like insulin to perform the same task of insulin in unlocking the doors of the cells of the body so that glucose can enter.

PANCREATIC TRANSPLANTATION

As alternatives to modification to insulin type and administration, research is active in replacing the failed pancreatic machinery for insulin production. Whole pancreas transplantation in Australia is usually performed in conjunction with transplantation of the kidney after kidney failure has occurred. Rejection of the kidney serves as an indicator of rejection of the pancreas, and so changes to immunosuppresive (anti-rejection) medications can be made more quickly. Although insulin secretion is not restored completely to normal, successful transplantation can free patients from the burden of blood glucose monitoring and insulin injections. The longer term outcome of the lessening and reversal of complications is not yet fully established.

Transplantation requires the use of immunosuppresive medications. These act to reduce the rejection capability of the immune system. Thus, they expose the patient to the risk of infection and, additionally, some worsen the diabetes. They are required because non-self tissue is recognised as being 'foreign' to the body, so such tissue is destroyed by the immune system (rejection). This hurdle is even greater with transplantation from animals (xenografts), although research continues into how to alter these grafts genetically so that the organ from an animal does not stimulate rejection by the human body.

Research into islet cell transplantation may yield an alternative to whole pancreatic transplantation, with the benefits of islet cells being able to be modified (outside the body prior to transplantation) so that they are rendered non-immunogenic (not recognised as being foreign). Otherwise, islet cells would also be destroyed by the same abnormal immune response which led to the development of insulin dependent diabetes mellitus (IDDM) initially. If only cells are transplanted, the transplantion procedure itself would be markedly simplified, and able to be done under local anaesthesia. Sources of islet cells include foetal tissue which has not developed the markers which identify the tissue as being foreign or modified animal islet cells. Ethical issues raised by these various transplantation procedures need to be considered.

MANAGEMENT AND PREVENTION OF COMPLICATIONS

In people with established diabetes mellitus, research is targeting improved means of preventing and treating complications. The past 10 years have seen the introduction of specific treatment for preventing and retarding the onset of kidney complications (nephropathy), and the widespread and effective use of laser photocoagulation for the management of eye problems (retinopathy). Trials of agents for the treatment of nerve damage (neuropathy) have so far been disappointing.

The management of arterial complications (large blood vessel disease) has been hampered by a lack of understanding of why atherosclerotic processes are so accelerated in diabetes. Better control of blood pressure is, however, recognised as being beneficial in lessening heart disease, stroke and kidney disease. The role of hormone replacement therapy (HRT) in diabetic women is currently being investigated as a means of reducing arterial disease.

PREVENTION

Non-insulin dependent diabetes mellitus (NIDDM)

As previously discussed, patients with NIDDM frequently have a lack of insulin relative to their bodies' requirements. This occurs because of insulin resistance, i.e. insulin cannot act effectively so more is needed to achieve the same blood glucose lowering effect.

This problem is not well tackled with current treatments, except with exercise and weight loss, which are effective means of reducing insulin resistance. Mechanisms of insulin resistance are not well understood and this is an area of active research. Some drugs that reduce insulin resistance are under trial at present.

Further knowledge is needed of the biochemical pathways involved in insulin interacting with its receptor to cause the entry of glucose into the cell. This would advance understanding of the mechanisms of insulin resistance and enable the design of treatment to reverse this metabolic defect. It would not only provide alternate treatments for NIDDM, but also possibly lead to means of preventing NIDDM, hypertension, dyslipidaemia and atherosclerosis.

Insulin dependent diabetes mellitus (IDDM)

As discussed in chapter 1, IDDM results from an abnormal immune response directed against the beta cell. This abnormal immune response begins several months or years prior to the onset of clinical IDDM. The pre-clinical or 'pre-diabetic' phase provides a window of opportunity to intervene and stop the progression to IDDM. Such people can be identified by antibodies (immune proteins) directed against various antigens (cell marker proteins) of the beta cell (e.g. islet cell antibodies, anti-insulin antibodies or glutamic acid decarboxylase antibodies) in conjuction with certain patterns of markers on their immune cells (HLA antigens).

Various agents have been tried and are undergoing trial as preventive agents in people who have been identified as being at risk of developing IDDM. Paradoxically, low-dose insulin given prior to the development of IDDM may prevent progression to IDDM. The difficulty in predicting accurately if a person is at risk of IDDM, together with the side effects of some of the preventive agents, hampers progress in this area. Immune intervention once IDDM is established is too late, since almost all of the beta cells have been destroyed. Prevention of IDDM in future may also involve immunisation against environmental triggers (such as particular viruses) of the abnormal immune response.

Conclusion

This book has been designed with the aim of supplementing the information that a person with diabetes, their family and friends may have already obtained from their health care providers. We look forward to future editions containing new information as researchers gain more knowledge into the cause and prevention of diabetes until the elimination of diabetes is finally achieved; the target at which we are all aiming.

With the realisation that the incidence of most of the potentially devastating complications of diabetes can be reduced through good glycaemic control has come a change in management of diabetes. Empowerment of the person with diabetes, with a sound knowledge base, places him or her in a better position to deal with a condition whose daily management interacts with all aspects of life.

Resources

This chapter helps with current addresses and phone and/or fax numbers for contacting diabetes associations and other useful groups in Australia and overseas.

DIABETES AUSTRALIA

Diabetes Australia is a consumer organisation which has provided a service to people with diabetes since 1937. This organisation has a National office in Canberra, but the services provided are largely decentralised with substantial provision of services by each state. Diabetes Australia publishes a quarterly magazine, *Diabetes Conquest*.

Throughout Australia a National Diabetes Supply Scheme (NDSS) is organised through Diabetes Australia. This scheme allows, at a subsidised price, the provision of blood and urine testing strips, and syringes or insulin pens or needles. There is no cost to enrolling in this scheme. The method of obtaining supplies differs in the various states. Usually supplies are available through a mail order system from Diabetes Australia, and/or in some states through pharmacies, acting as agents for Diabetes Australia.

>Diabetes Australia — National Office
>1st floor, Churchhill House
>218 Northbourne Ave
>Braddon, ACT 2612
>Tel: (02) 6230 1155
>Fax: (02) 6230 1535

Australian Capital Territory:
Diabetes Australia — ACT
PO Box 3727
Western Creek ACT 2611
Tel: (02) 6288 9830
Fax: (02) 6257 6046

New South Wales: Diabetes Australia — NSW
26 Arundel St
Glebe NSW 2037
(GPO Box 9824, Sydney NSW 2001)
Tel: (02) 9660 3200
Fax: (02) 9660 3633

Queensland: Diabetes Australia — Qld
Cnr Ernest & Merivale Sts
SOUTH BRISBANE QLD 4101
(PO Box 3814, South Brisbane Qld 4101)
Tel: (07) 3846 4600
Fax: (07) 3846 4642

Northern Territory: Diabetes Australia — NT
2 Tiwi Place
Tiwi NT 0810
(GPO Box 40113, Casuarina NT 0811)
Tel: (08) 8927 8488/ 8927 8482
Fax: (08) 8927 8515

Western Australia: Diabetes Australia — WA
48 Wickham St
East Perth WA 6000
(PO Box 6097, East Perth WA 6004)
Tel: (08) 9325 7699
Fax: (08) 9221 1183

South Australia: Diabetes Australia — SA
159 Burbridge Rd (Unit 4)
Hilton SA 5033
(GPO Box 1930, Adelaide SA 5001)
Tel: (08) 8234 1977
Fax: (08) 8234 2013

Victoria: Diabetes Australia — Vic
3rd Floor, 100 Collins St
Melbourne VIC 3000
Tel: (03) 9654 8777
Fax: (03) 9650 1917

Tasmania: Diabetes Australia — Tas
79 Davey St
Hobart TAS 7000
Tel: (03) 6234 5223
Fax: (03) 6224 0105

Juvenile Diabetes Foundation Australia (JDFA)
JDFA is a consumer organisation specialising in providing support primarily to children and young adults with insulin dependent diabetes, and their families. JDFA, like Diabetes Australia, is a non-profit organisation. The primary objective of JDFA is to support and fund research aimed at finding a cure for diabetes. Address for JDFA is:

Juvenile Diabetes Foundation Australia
PO Box 1500
Chatswood NSW 2067
Tel: (02) 9411 4087
Fax: 9411 8905

Australian Diabetes Educators' Association (ADEA)
The ADEA promotes awareness of diabetes education and recognition of diabetes educators as a cornerstone of diabetes health care in hospitals and throughout the community.

Australian Diabetes Educators' Association
1st floor, East Wing, Churchhill House
218 Northbourne Ave
Braddon, ACT 2612
Tel: (02) 6230 1228
Fax: (02) 6230 1413

Dietitian Associations
National office: Dietitians Association of Australia
1/8 Phipps Cl
Deakin ACT 2600
Tel: (02) 6282 9555
Fax: (02) 6282 9888

New South Wales: Dietitians Association of Australia
232 Pitt St
Sydney NSW 2000
(PO Box A207, Sydney South 2000)
Tel: (02) 9267 2302
Fax: (02) 9267 2302

Queensland: Dietitians Association of Australia
PO Box 5069
Kenmore East QLD 4069
Tel: (0419) 797 428

Nothern Territory: Dietitians Association of Australia
PO Box 42570
Casuarina NT 0810
Tel: (08) 8973 8631

Western Australia: Dietitians Association of Australia
PO Box 226
West Perth WA 6872
Tel: (08) 9388 1486
Fax: (08) 9388 1492

South Australia: Dietitians Association of Australia
PO Box 204
North Adelaide SA 5006
Tel: (08) 8282 1211

Victoria: Dietitians Association of Australia
212 Clarendon St
East Melbourne VIC 3002
Tel: (03) 9419 0586
Fax: (03) 9386 3348

Tasmania: Dietitians Association of Australia
GPO Box 726
Hobart TAS 7001
Tel: (03) 6221 6475

Podiatry Associations

New South Wales: Australian Podiatry Association (NSW)
Suite 20/450 Elizabeth Street
Surry Hills NSW 2010
Tel: (02) 9698 3751
Fax: (02) 9698 7116

Queensland: Australian Podiatry Association (Qld)
PO Box 4066
Raceview QLD 4305
Tel/Fax: (07) 3282 7066

Western Australia: Australian Podiatry Association (WA)
6/20 Leura St
Nedlands WA 6009
Tel: (08) 9386 1560
Fax: (08) 9386 1550

South Australia: Australian Podiatry Association (SA)
8/15 Fullarton Rd
Kent Town SA 5067
Tel: (08) 8363 4144
Fax: (08) 8362 2223

Victoria: Australian Podiatry Association (Vic)
26/456 St Kilda Rd
Melbourne VIC 3004
Tel: (03) 9866 5906
Fax: (03) 9866 2094

Tasmania: Australian Podiatry Association (Tas)
75 Waverley St
Bellerive TAS 7018
Tel/Fax: (03) 6245 0588

Facilities for visually impaired

New South Wales: Royal Blind Society
4 Mitchell St
Enfield NSW 2135
(PO Box 176, Burwood NSW 2134)
Tel: (02) 9334 3333
Fax: (02) 9747 5993

Australian Capital Territory:
: Royal Blind Society
ACT & South East Reginal Office
Red Cross House
Cnr Hindmarsh Drive & Palmer St
Garran ACT 2605
Tel: (02) 6285 3344
Fax: (02) 6285 4900

Queensland:
: Royal Blind Society of Queensland
247 Vulture St
South Brisbane QLD 4101

34 Cleveland St
Stones Corner QLD 4120
Tel: (07) 3397 1234

Western Australia:
: Royal West Australian Institute for the Blind
134 Whatley Cres
(PO Box 14)
Maylands WA 6051
Tel: (08) 9272 1122
Fax: (08) 9272 6600

South Australia:
: Royal Society for the Blind of South Australia
Blacks Rd
Gilles Plains SA 5086
(PO Box 196, Greenacres, SA 5086)
Tel: (08) 261 4611
Client Information Line (08) 261 4623

Branches:
: Adelaide Low Vision Centre
Knapman House
230 Pirie St
Adelaide SA 5000
Tel: (08) 8232 4777
Fax: (08) 8232 2111

Victoria:	Royal Victorian Institute for the Blind
557 St Kilda Rd
Melbourne VIC 3004
Tel: (03) 9529 3544
Fax: (03) 9510 4735

Tasmania:	Royal Tasmanian Society for the Blind
& Deaf
164 Elizabeth St
Hobart TAS 7000
Tel: (03) 6234 3077

Diabetes Associations in other countries

Argentina:	Sociedad Argentina de Diabetes
Argentinian Diabetes Society
Piso 8, Dolo 74
Calle Paraguay 1307, 8 71
1057 Buenos Aires
Argentina
Tel: 54-1/42-84-19
Fax: 54-1/813-84-19

Belgium:	Association Belge du Diabete
Belgian Diabetes Association
Chaussee de Waterloo 935
1180 Bruxelles
Belgium
Tel: 32-2/374-31-95
Fax: 32-2/374-81-74

Brazil:	Sociedade Brasiliera de Daibetes (SBD)
Brazilian Diabetes Society
av. Paulista 2073 - Edif. Horsa I-ej2123
01311-300 Sao Paulo
Brazil
Tel:/Fax: 55-11/289-2941

Canada:	Canadian Diabetes Association
15 Toronto Street, Suite 1001
Toronto, Ontario, M5C 2E3
Canada
Tel: 1-416/363-0177 ext 475
Fax: 1-416/363-3393

China:	Chinese Diabetes Society of the Chinese Medical Association (CMA) Department of Diabetes Research Huashan Hospital Shanghai Medical University Shanghai 200040 Peoples Republic of China Tel: 86-21/6248-9999 Fax: 86-21/6248-9191
England:	British Diabetic Association 10 Queen Anne Street London WIM OBD United Kingdom Tel: 44-171/323-1531 Fax: 44-171/637-3644
Fiji:	Fiji National Diabetes Foundation CWM Hospital GPO Box 115 Suva, Fiji Tel: 679/313-444 Fax: 679/303-232
France:	Association Francaise des Diabetiques 58 rue Alexandre Dumas 75544 Paris Cedex 11 France Tel: 33-1/40-09-24-25 Fax: 33-1/40-09-20-30
Germany:	Deutsche Diabetes Union e.V. German Diabetes Union Drosselweg 16 82152 Krailling Germany Tel: 49-89/857-1249 Fax: 49-89/857-6488

Hong Kong:	Diabetic Division, Society for the Study of Endocrinology, Metabolism & Reproduction Suite 813, Central Building 1-3 Pedder Street Central Hong Kong Hong Kong Tel: 852/2523-2662 Fax: 852/2525-6472
India:	Diabetic Association of India Raheja Hospital Road Mahim - Bombay 400016 Tel: 91-22/27 38 13 Fax: 91-22/649-8569
Indonesia: (PERSADI)	Persatuan Diabetes Indonesia Indonesian Diabetes Association Jalan Geusan Ulun No17 Bandung 40115 Indonesia Tel: 62/22-438-251 Fax: 62/22-436-461
Israel:	Israel Diabetes Association Jaborinsky 42 Givatim 50318 Israel Tel: 972-3/573-2445 Fax: 972-3/731-9796
Italy:	Associazione Italiana Diabetici via Dracone 23 20126 Milano Italy Tel/Fax: 39-2/257-01-76

Japan:	Japan Diabetes Society
Hongo Sky Building 403
3-38-11 Hongo 3-chome
Bunkyo-ku Tokyo 113
Japan
Tel: 81-3-3/815-4364
Fax: 81-3-3/815-7985

New Zealand:	Diabetes New Zealand, Inc.
1 Coquet Street
PO Box 54
Oamaru 8915, South Island
New Zealand
Tel: 64-3/434-8110
Fax: 64-3/434-5281

Singapore:	Diabetic Society of Singapore
Ang Mo Kio Community Hospital
17 Ang Mo Kio Avenue 9 - 02-12
Republic of Singapore 569766
Tel: 65/450-6132
Fax: 65/553-1801

South Africa:	South African Diabetes Association
PO Box 1715
Saxonwold 2132
South Africa
Tel: 27-21/447-6265
Fax: 27-21/447-5100

Sweden:	Svenska Diabetes Forbundet
Swedish Diabetes Association
PO Box 1545
171 29 Solna
Sweden
Tel: 46-8/629-8580, Fax: 46-8/98-2535

United States of America:
American Diabetes Association
1660 Duke Street
Alexandria, VA 22314
United States of America
Tel: 1-703/549-1500
Fax: 1-703/683-1839

Glossary

Amino acids Amino acids are the building blocks of which the body's proteins are made. These proteins are necessary for metabolism and growth.

Antigen Substance or part of a substance that is recognised as being foreign and so the body produces an immune response (antibodies) against the antigen. Antigens can be made in the body or introduced into the body.

Carbohydrate These are a class of chemical compounds composed of carbon, hydrogen and oxygen. This includes starches and sugars. Carbohydrates are the preferred fuel for the body.

Claudication Severe pain felt in the calves during walking, often relieved by rest. The pain is a result of poor blood supply to the muscle.

Dyslipidaemia A situation where there is a disorder of the levels of fats in the blood e.g. as in the case of too much cholesterol.

Enzymes Complex proteins able to induce chemical changes in other substances without being changed themselves.

Fats Fats are a concentrated form of storing energy. Also known as lipids.

Fibre The indigestible part of the foods humans eat. Also known as 'roughage'. Only found in cereals, vegetables and fruit.

Fluorescein angiography Following an injection of radiopaque dye, x-rays are taken of the blood vessels at the back of the eyes.

Glycaemic index A measure of the effect of an individual food on the blood glucose level.

Immunosuppressive Acting to suppress the body's natural immune response to an antigen.

Impotence When an adult male is unable to achieve erection of the penis.

Insulin receptor An area on the cell wall with which insulin reacts allowing glucose to pass into the cell.

Interstitium (Interstitial). Placed in spaces between tissues or within organs.

Kilojoule Metric measurement of energy (also known as the calorie). This is the imperial measurement of energy. Has been replaced by the kilojoule (1 calorie = 4.186 kilojoules).

Minerals Inorganic elements necessary for the normal functioning of the human body. At least 20 minerals are known to be essential for health.

Monounsaturated fats A type of fat with only one incomplete chemical bond in their structure. Found in all fats, but high in olive, canola and macadamia nut oils.

Neovascularisation (vascularisation) The development of new tiny blood vessels in a tissue.

Oral glucose tolerance test A diagnostic test to find out if a person has diabetes. After a fasting blood glucose levels is taken, a standard dose of glucose is given in a drink. The blood glucose is again measured at half hourly intervals over the next 2 hours.

Organogenesis Refers to the formation of a baby's organs during the first 8 weeks of the mother's pregnancy.

Osteoporosis A disorder where the bones are weakened due to being more porous.

Osteoarthritis A chronic degenerative disease of the joints especially joints that bear the weight of the body. There is often pain and limitation of movement.

Peptide A compound made up of two or more amino acids.

Polyunsaturated fats A type of fat with 2 or more incomplete chemical bonds in their structure. Found in: vegetable and nut oils, e.g. sunflower, peanut, maize etc, polyunsaturated margarines and fish.

Portal circulation Circulation of blood to the liver from the digestive tract, pancreas, spleen and gallbladder.

Protein Essential nutrient for growth, maintenance and renewal of body tissue.

Saturated fats A type of fat with no incomplete chemical bonds. Found mostly in animal fats. However, palm and coconut oils are also mainly saturated fat.

Stillbirth or stillborn This refers to the birth of a foetus who died either before or during delivery.

Vitamins Organic elements essential to the normal functioning of the body. The majority of these cannot be made by the body and must be obtained from food. Found in very small quantities in most foods.

INDEX

acarbose, 80
ACE inhibitor, 100
acesulphame potassium, 46, 169
activity,
  see exercise
acute (short term) diabetic complications,
  see hyperglycaemia, 89
  hyperosmolar coma, 153
  hypoglycaemia, 81
  ketoacidosis, 91
adolescence, 148-152
  challenges, 149-150
  tips on survival, 150-152
aerobic exercise, 54
alcohol, 29, 164, 167
American Diabetes Association, 198
anaerobic exercise, 55
Argentinian Diabetes Association, 195
arteriosclerosis (thickened arteries), 101
  prevention, 101
  treatment, 101
artificial sweetener 46, 169
aspartame, 46, 169
atherosclerosis (large vessel disease), 13, 100
Australian Dietary Guidelines, 26-30
Australian Podiatry Association, 109, 193
autonomic neuropathy (nerve damage), 103

barrier methods (contraception), 118
basal bolus regimen, 67
Belgian Diabetes Association, 195
beta cells, 3, 184
biguanide, 73
  action, 74
  side effects, 74
blood glucose, 16-22
  acceptable range, 9, 17
  frequency of testing, 20
  monitoring, 14, 17-22
  normal range, 3, 9, 19
  timing of tests, 20
blood glucose meters, 19
blurred vision, 4
Brazilian Diabetes Society, 195
British Diabetic Association, 196

calcium, 26, 30
calluses and corns, 106
Canadian Diabetes Association, 195
carbohydrate, 25, 28, 36, 40, 42-46
cataracts (opaqueness lens of the eye), 12, 98
  prevention, 99
  treatment, 99,
Chinese Diabetes Society, 196
cholesterol (a blood fat), 28, 37-38, 40, 48
Code of Practice (re food labels), 35
combination therapy, 79
complications of diabetes, *see*
  acute (short term), 89
  long term, 96
  prevention, 96
contraception, 118
contraception methods, 118
cooking tips for health, 48-50
corns and calluses, 106
coronary artery disease, 12, 13, 101
cutting toe nails, 105
cyclamate, 46, 169

Diabetes Australia, 21, 189
Diabetes Control and Complication Trial, 13, 15
Diabetes mellitus 1
  characteristics, 1-7
  definition, 3-5
  diagnosis, 5-6
  gestational, 115, 116
  in adolescence, 148-152
  in pregnancy, 110-117
  in the elderly, 153-161
  treatment, 8-15
  types, 3-5
diabetic ketoacidosis, 5, 92

diabetic nephropathy
  (kidney disease),   12,13,99
  prevention,   99
  treatment,   99
diabetic retinopathy (diabetic
  eye disease),   12,13,97
  prevention,   98
  treatment,   98
diagnosis of diabetes,   5
diet/dietary,   23-50
  principles of diabetic diet, 23, 26
Dietitians Association of
  Australia,   23, 191
dinner parties and other
  celebrations,   165-166

eating out,   162-169
elderly person with diabetes,
    153-161
  aims of treatment,   154-159
  education,   155
  nutrition,   155-156
  prevention of complications,
    154, 159-161
energy (food related),   23-24
exercise,
    28, 31-32, 51-57, 70, 156-157
  adjusting food/medication,   56
  effects of exercise in
    diabetes,   33, 52
  monitoring blood glucose
    levels,   55
  types,   54

facilities for visually impaired
  people,   193-195
fat (in food),
    24-25, 28, 36-41, 163-164
fat atrophy/hypertrophy,   61
feet, see foot
fertility,   110
fibre,   25, 36-37, 47, 199
Fiji National Diabetes
  Foundation,   196
food label reading,   34-37, 39
foot   104
  assessment,   105
  complications,   102
  first aid,   107
  routine care,   104
footwear,   107-108
French Diabetes Association, 196

fructosamine,   21

German Diabetes Union,   196
gestational diabetes,   115
  diagnosis,   116
  effects on baby and
    mother,   116-117
  screening,   116
glaucoma,   161
glucagon,   86-87
  how to inject,   87
  indications for use,   87
  what it is,   86-87
glucose tolerance test (GTT),
  see oral glucose tolerance test
glycemic index,   42-44, 199
glycosylated haemoglobin 16,21

HbA1c, see glycosylated
  haemoglobin
health insurance companies, 171
health professionals,   171
heart disease,   101
heredity,   6
hidden fats (in food),   39-41
high blood pressure, see
  hypertension
hormone replacement
  therapy,   118, 120
hyperglycaemia (high blood
  glucose),   89
  causes,   89-90
  definition,   89
  how to treat,   91
  symptoms,   90
hyperosmolar coma,   153-154
hypertension (high blood
  pressure),   100
  prevention,   100
  treatment,   100
hypoglycaemia (low blood
  glucose),   81
  causes,   82-83
  definition,   81
  how to treat,   84-86
  prevention,   87-88
  symptoms,   81-82
hypoglycaemic unawareness,   84

IDDM, see insulin dependent
  diabetes mellitus
Indian Diabetes Association, 197

Index

Indonesian Diabetes
  Association, 197
insulin (produced in the body) 2-3
  action, 2, 87
insulin (manufactured) 65-67, 76
  action, 66
  adjustment of dose, 68
  administration, 64
  drawing up, 62
  insulin pens, 59
  insulin pumps, 60
  insulin syringes, 58
  injecting, 60
  mixing, 63
  regimen, 67, 78, 79
  storage, 61
  types, 65, 78, 79
Insulin dependent diabetes
  mellitus (IDDM),
    3, 6, 65, 111, 187
insulin resistance, 3
insurance, 171
  health, 171
  travel, 176
intermediate acting insulin,
    66, 67, 70
intrauterine device
  (contraception), 119
iron (food related), 30
isomalt, 46,169
Israel Diabetes Association, 197
Italian Diabetes Association, 197

Japan Diabetes Society, 198
Juvenile Diabetes Foundation
  Australia, 191
Juvenile onset diabetes, see
  Insulin
  dependent diabetes mellitus,

ketoacidosis, 5, 91-92
  see diabetic ketoacidosis
  causes, 92
  prevention, 92
  symptoms, 92
ketones, 5, 7, 17, 91,92
ketonuria, 16,17
kidney disease, see diabetic
  nephropathy

laser therapy (for eyes), 98
leg circulation, impairment of 101

lens, 98
life insurance, 171
long acting insulin, 66, 67
long term complications, 96
  cataracts, 98
  checklist on complication
    prevention, 96
  eye 'retina' damage, 97
  kidney damage, 99
  heart disease, 101
  nerve damage, 102
  poor blood circulation, 101

maturity onset diabetes, see
  non-insulin
  dependent diabetes mellitus
maturity onset diabetes of the
  young, 4
medical investigations and
  operations, 94
meters, see blood glucose meters
metformin, 73, 74
microalbumin test, 99
minerals (food related), 24,26,28
mixing insulin, 63
monounsaturated fats, 200

National Diabetes Supply
  Scheme, 21-22, 189
nephropathy, see diabetic
  nephropathy
New Zealand Diabetes Inc. 198
neuropathy (nerve damage), 102
  autonomic, 103
  peripheral, 102
Non-insulin dependent diabetes
  mellitus (NIDDM),
    4-6, 72, 78, 79, 186
nutrition, 23-30
nutrition claims, 34-37

oral contraceptives, 119
oral glucose tolerance test, 200
oral hypoglycaemic agents, 73
overweight or obesity, 30-33
  causes, 28,31
  treatments, 31-33
pancreatic transplants, 185-186
pens, insulin 59
peripheral neuropathy (nerve
  damage), 102
  prevention, 103

treatment, 103
podiatrist, role of 108
polydextrose 46, 169
polyunsaturated fats, 24-25, 38
pregnancy, *see* gestational diabetes, diabetes in pregnancy,
pre-mixed insulin 67
pre-pregnancy management, 113
protein (food related), 24, 200
psychological effects of diabetes, 140
psychological health, 10

relaxation therapy, 145-147
renal threshold, 17
research in diabetes, 184-187
retinopathy (diabetic eye disease), 98
Road Traffic Authority, 170-171
role of the podiatrist, 108
role of relaxation, 145-146
Royal Blind Society, 193

saccharin, 46
salt 29, 37
saturated fat, 24-25, 28, 38, 39
sexual changes, 130-131
   age related, 130
   with diabetes, 129-130
sexual difficulties, men 128
   ejaculatory difficulties, 134
   erectile difficulties, 134
   inhibited/retarded ejaculation, 135-136
   painful ejaculation, 137
   retrograde/dry ejaculation, 136-137
sexual difficulties, women 129
   painful intercourse, 138
   orgasmic difficulty, 137-138
   vaginismus, 138-139
sexuality, 121-139
   communication about sex, 131
   normal development, 125
   myths, 122
sexual response changes with diabetes, 130-131
sexual response cycle, 125
short acting insulin, 66, 67
Singapore Diabetic Society, 198
smoking, 96

sodium, *see* salt
South African Diabetes Association, 198
stress, 140-147
   effects of stress, 141
   sources of stress, 142
stress hormones, 93, 140
stress management, 141
   principles of management, 141-145
stress reaction, 140
stroke, 101
sucralose, 46
sugar, dietary 25, 29, 36-37, 42-43, 47, 163
sulphonylureas, 73-75
   action, 75
   side effects, 75
Swedish Diabetes Association, 198
symptoms of diabetes, 90
syringes, 58

takeaway foods, 162, 164-165
testing (self), 17
   blood glucose level, 19
   urine ketones, 16
thiazolidinediones, 80
tinea (fungal infection), 106
toe nail cutting, 105
travel and diabetes, 174-183
   first aid kit, 182-183
   insurance, 176
   preparations, 175
travel and illness, 181-182
triglycerides (blood fat), 48
tubal ligation (contraception), 119
Type 1 diabetes, *see* Insulin dependent diabetes mellitus,
Type 2 diabetes, *see* Non-insulin dependent diabetes mellitus,

ulcers (foot), 104
urine testing, 16
   glucose, 16
   ketones, 16, 17

vasectomy (contraception), 119
very short acting insulin, 66, 70
vitamins, 24, 25-26, 28, 200
vomiting, 93-94